D0056909

Main

The
Brain
Warrior's
Way

The
Brain
Warrior's
Way

Ignite Your Energy and Focus
Attack Illness and Aging
Transform Pain into Purpose

DANIEL G. AMEN, MD
TANA AMEN, BSN, RN

NEW AMERICAN LIBRARY
NEW YORK

NEW AMERICAN LIBRARY
Published by Berkley
An imprint of Penguin Random House LLC
375 Hudson Street, New York, New York 10014

Library of Congress Cataloging-in-Publication Data
Names: Amen, Daniel G. | Amen, Tana.
Title: The brain warrior's way: ignite your energy and focus, attack illness and aging, transform pain into purpose/Daniel G. Amen, MD, Tana Amen, BSN, RN.
Description: First edition. | New York: New American Library, 2016.
Identifiers: LCCN 2016028440 (print) | LCCN 2016040980 (ebook) | ISBN 9781101988473 | ISBN 9781101988497 (ebook)
Subjects: LCSH: Self-care, Health—Popular works. | Mental health—Popular works. | Stress management—Popular works. | Mental health—Nutritional aspects—Popular works.
Classification: LCC RA776.95 .A4595 2016 (print) | LCC RA776.95 (ebook) | DDC 613—dc23
LC record available at https://lccn.loc.gov/2016028440

First Edition: November 2016

Printed in the United States of America
3   5   7   9   10   8   6   4   2

Jacket design by Steve Meditz
Book design by Pauline Neuwirth

To Chloe, Eli, Emmy, Liam, and Louie and the rest of our tribe—our reasons for being Brain Warriors.

Contents

The Brain Warrior's Way

◼

A warrior is someone who is committed to master oneself
at all levels, who develops the courage to do the right
thing for yourself, others, and community.

—*THE WAY OF THE SEAL* BY MARK DIVINE

T HE WAR FOR YOUR HEALTH is won or lost between your ears,
in the moment-by-moment decisions your brain makes every day.
When your brain works right your decisions are much more likely to be
effective and add laserlike focus, energy, and health to your life. When your
brain is troubled, for whatever reason, you are much more likely to make
bad decisions that steal your energy, focus, moods, memory, and health and
lead to your early destruction and trouble in future generations.

Bushido (Japanese: "way of the warrior") is the code of ethics for the
samurai. It is a way of living that is required to be a warrior. Samurais
ascribe to a culture focused on constant, never-ending self-improvement
in an effort to protect themselves and those they love. The Brain Warrior's Way is also a way of living, a clear path we have developed over
three decades of helping tens of thousands of patients at Amen Clinics
have better brains and better lives. In addition, we have used this path
to help people in the military, businesses, churches, schools, and drug
rehabilitation centers. Living the Brain Warrior's Way will improve your
decision-making ability and sense of personal power and help your

- Energy
- Focus
- Moods
- Memory

- Weight
- Relationships
- Work
- Overall health

The Brain Warrior's Way is a unique and powerful program and the only one of its kind to improve the health of your brain and body. It is grounded in scientific research and designed to help you live with vitality, a clear mind and excellent health—even if you are struggling or are in pain right now—even if you've made unhealthy choices for many years. This program will help you turn your health around. Don't you want to wake up feeling good inside and out every day?

By following the Brain Warrior's Way, you will transform the health of not just your brain and body, but the brains and bodies of those you love and care for. The new science of epigenetics has taught us that your habits turn on or off certain genes that make illnesses and early death more or less likely in you, and also in your children and grandchildren. The war for the health of your brain and body is not just about you. It is about generations of you.

Step by step, this book will show you how to develop a Brain Warrior's MASTERY over your physical and mental health. It will teach you:

Mind-set of a Brain Warrior—knowing your motivation to be healthy and focusing on abundance, never deprivation

Assessment of a Brain Warrior—having a clear strategy, brain health assessment, knowing and optimizing your important numbers, fighting the war on multiple fronts, and always being on the lookout to prevent future trouble

Sustenance of a Brain Warrior—knowing the food and supplements that fuel success and give you a competitive edge

Training of a Brain Warrior—engaging in the daily habits and routines that protect your health

Essence of a Brain Warrior—transforming your pain into passion and knowing why the world is a better place because you are here

Responsibilities of a Brain Warrior—taking the critical step of sharing information and creating your own tribe of Brain Warriors

Yearlong Basic Training of a Brain Warrior—making lasting changes with tools that will last a lifetime

- Serious
- Purposeful
- Informed
- Aware
- Prepared
- Nourished

- Highly trained
- Deeply honest
- Passionate
- Protective
- Relentless

Along the way you will meet dozens of triumphant Brain Warriors who were once prisoners of the war for their health. Their stories will inspire and encourage you into a new way of living.

BRAIN WARRIOR BILL

Here is a note from the leader of an East Coast Young Presidents' Organization (YPO) Pod whose group spent three days with us at Amen Clinics learning the principles of the Brain Warrior's Way.

> *"The program dramatically changed my life, allowing me to lose weight, and to focus unlike I could ever remember. My depression faded away and my focus and productivity improved. As a group, we universally agreed that the visit to Amen Clinics had the greatest impact on our lives in over a decade of being together."*

Most people don't want to think about wars and warriors, and we would prefer not to either, but if you open your eyes and tell yourself the truth about what is happening in our society it is painfully obvious: we are in a war for the health of our brains and bodies. Americans die younger and experience more illness than people in other wealthy nations, despite spending nearly twice as much on health care per person.[1] Close to 75 percent of our health-care dollars are spent on chronic *preventable* illnesses, including Alzheimer's disease, depression, ADD/ADHD, diabetes and prediabetes, and obesity.

WHY WE ARE IN A WAR FOR OUR HEALTH

And this is not just an adult war. Huge corporations are targeting your children and grandchildren. When a clown or a king with a billion-dollar bankroll can come into your living room and bribe your children with toys to get them to eat low-quality, nonnutritious foods that promote illness and early death it's time to fight back. According to a recent study, the toys fast-food companies use to entice children are highly effective weapons in hooking their developing brains to want more of what will hurt their health.[2] In addition, well-meaning organizations, such as the Girl Scouts, enlist young girls to sell unhealthful cookies as a way to fund their activities, and few people think twice about the sugar, vegetable oil, partially hydrogenated fats, and artificial preservatives that promote disease.

You are in a war for your health. Nearly everywhere you go (schools, work, shopping malls, movie theaters, airports, ball parks, and so on), someone is trying to sell you food that will kill you early. The standard American diet (SAD) is filled with pro-inflammatory foods that increase your risk for diabetes, hypertension, heart disease, cancer, ADHD, depression, and dementia.[3] It is also associated with a smaller hippocampus, one of the major memory structures in the brain.[4]

The real weapons of mass destruction in our society are foods that are

- Highly processed
- Pesticide sprayed
- Artificially colored and sweetened
- High glycemic
- Low fiber
- Foodlike substances
- Laden with hormones
- Tainted with antibiotics

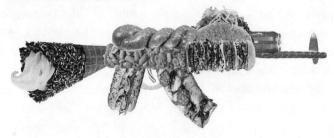

Plus the companies that produce these unhealthful foods not only use toys to hook tiny human brains but also use neuroscience tricks to hijack adult brains. They purposefully associate gorgeous, scantily clad women with poor-quality food to hook your pleasure centers, somehow getting you to make the illogical connection that if you eat those foods, either these women will want you or you will look like them. You must know there's no way these beautiful women would look the way they do if their diet regularly consisted of cheeseburgers that dripped mayonnaise, mustard, and ketchup down their blouses.

In addition, many corporations brag about the addictive nature of their foods, "Bet you can't eat just one." They hire food scientists to combine fat, sugar, and salt with the perfect texture, crunchiness, meltiness, and aroma to overwhelm the brain with flavor to trigger the "bliss point" in your brain, which is akin to taking a hit of cocaine, making you literally fall in love with low-quality foods. This is one of the reasons people say they love candy, doughnuts, pastries, french fries, and bread and can't ever conceive of giving them up. They are not eating to live; they are eating to feed addictions that were artificially created for a profit motive. We had one woman tell us she would rather get cancer than give up sugar. We wondered aloud if she dated the bad boys in high school. Being in love with something that hurts you is a position that needs some serious reexamination.

No food of any kind belongs in the same emotional place in your brain as the love you have for your spouse, children, or grandchildren. Many ancient warriors considered dependence on anything, especially food, a weakness, and totally unacceptable. They ate to win; their survival depended on it. We want you to do the same thing if you truly love yourself, your health, your loved ones, and future generations.

The war for your health is not just about our modern-day adulterated food. News outlets repeatedly pour toxic thoughts into our brains, making us see terror or disaster around every corner to boost their ratings. The constant frightening images activate our brains' primitive fear circuits (amygdala) that once ensured our survival but are now obsolete. The news always highlights the sensational, evil, and most awful stories to keep you hooked to their channels or websites. Unless you purposefully monitor your news intake, these companies succeed in raising your stress hormones, which over time shrink the major memory centers in your brain and put excessive fat around your waist—and belly fat is particularly toxic, because it converts healthy testosterone into unhealthy, cancer-promoting forms of estrogen. Do you reach for your phone first thing in the morning to see what awful things have happened in the world overnight? You might not have known that this habit is adversely affecting your health, but now you do.

You are in a war for your health. It is further fueled by technology companies that are constantly creating addictive gadgets that hook our attention and distract us from meaningful relationships.[5] Many people are on their phones at mealtimes, rather than interacting with family members. A 2015 study found that teens actually spend more time on social media (average 9 hours) than they do asleep. Tweens are online 6 hours a day.[6] Technology has hijacked developing brains with potentially serious consequences for many.

At Amen Clinics we have treated many teens and adults with video game or pornography addictions. One teenager became violent whenever his parents limited his play. We scanned his brain while he played video games and then later after he had abstained from playing any games for a month. It was like we were looking at the brains of two different people. The video games caused abnormal firing in his left temporal lobe, an area of the brain often associated with violence. When he was off video games, he was one of the sweetest, most polite young men we had met; but when on them, it was a completely different story.

Daniel did a Tinder experiment for the *Dr. Oz Show* using brain scans to see the effect of the dating site on mood and focus. He demonstrated that, in some individuals, the dating site can make people more vulnerable to anxiety and depression.

As video game and technology usage goes up, so do obesity and depression.[7] Ian Bogost, famous video game designer (*Cow Clicker* and *Cruel 2 B Kind*) and chair of media studies and professor of interactive computing at the Georgia Institute of Technology, calls the wave of new habit-forming technologies "the cigarettes of this century" and warns of their equally addictive and potentially destructive side effects.[8]

As part of the gadget revolution, disturbing new research from Microsoft reported that humans lose concentration after about 8 seconds, while the lowly goldfish loses its focus after about 9 seconds.[9] It seems like evolution may be going in the wrong direction. In 2000, the human attention span average was estimated at 12 seconds, which is not great; but losing a third of our attention span in fifteen years is alarming!

According to an article in *Harvard Business Review*, "Beware of the Busy Manager," our unhealthful lifestyles are diminishing our capacity at work.[10] Only 10 percent of managers score high in both focus and energy, two of the main ingredients for success. The authors found that 20 percent of managers were disengaged, 30 percent scored high in procrastination, and 40 percent were easily distracted. This means that 90 percent of managers, and likely the rest of us, lack focus and/or energy.

These and other assaults on our brains and bodies have potentially devastating long-term consequences.

THE CONSEQUENCES OF THE WAR
FOR OUR HEALTH

Genes play a more minor role than you might think, and many diseases are born out of unhealthful choices and behaviors, regardless of whether there is a genetic predisposition. Sadly, all around us we can see the devastating consequences of preventable illness.

Alzheimer's disease is expected to triple by 2050, and there is no cure on the horizon. Alzheimer's disease affects 50 percent of people age eighty-five and older. If you are fortunate to live until you are eighty-five or beyond you have a one-in-two chance of losing your mind along the way. To make matters worse, recent brain-imaging research has demonstrated that Alzheimer's disease and other forms of dementia actually start in the brain decades before you have any symptoms. Below is a brain SPECT scan, which measures blood flow and activity, of a fifty-nine-year-old woman diagnosed with Alzheimer's disease compared to someone with a healthy brain. You can see the back half of her brain is deteriorating. She likely had trouble in her brain in her thirties or forties.

Premature cognitive impairment leads to diminished work performance, which can lead to hardships among a workforce that grows older every year. With people working longer than ever before, even minor drops in brain function can jeopardize your productivity and job security. Since the 2008 recession, the average retirement age has risen from age fifty-seven to age sixty-two and by 2020 it is estimated that 25 percent of American workers will be fifty-five or older. The exciting news is that new research suggests that you can decrease your risk of Alzheimer's disease and other forms of dementia by 60 percent or more, and those same strategies will help your mood, focus, and memory. The Brain Warrior's Way will clearly lay out those strategies for you.

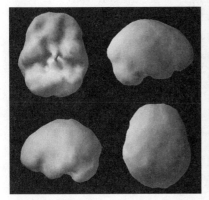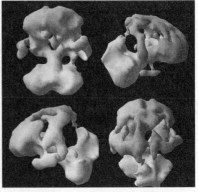

Healthy
Full, even, symmetrical activity

Alzheimer's
Decreased activity in back of brain

Depression is one of the greatest killers of our time. It affects 50 million Americans at some point in their lives and has increased 400 percent since 1987. Depression is associated with suicide, divorce, job failure, heart disease, obesity, and dementia. Depression doubles the risk of Alzheimer's disease in women and quadruples it in men. A staggering 23 percent of women between the ages of twenty and sixty are taking antidepressant medications. The risk of depression also significantly increases after the age of sixty-five.[11]

Attention deficit disorder (ADD), also called attention deficit hyperactivity disorder (ADHD), is now being diagnosed more frequently than ever. Statistics from the Centers for Disease Control and Prevention (CDC) report that nearly one in five high-school-age boys and 11 percent of school-age children overall have received a diagnosis of ADD, including an estimated 6.4 million children between the ages of six and seventeen. This is a 16 percent increase since 2007 and a 41 percent increase in the past decade.[12] This rapid rise of ADD is due to many factors, including low-fat, low-fiber, high-glycemic diets; increased use of electronics; decreased exercise; and diminished sleep. Many people underestimate the devastating consequences of ADD. Yet, when left untreated, it is associated with school underachievement and failure (35 percent never finish high school), drug and alcohol abuse (according to one study from Harvard, 52 percent of untreated ADD adults have a substance abuse problem), job failure, divorce, incarceration, obesity, depression, and dementia.

Diabetes or prediabetes now affects 50 percent of the U.S. population, according to a 2015 study published in the *Journal of the American Medical*

Association.[13] Blood sugar problems have dramatically escalated in the last thirty years. In 1960, one out of a hundred people in America had type 2 diabetes; today that ratio has changed to one out of ten people, a tenfold increase. Since the 1980s, the rate of type 2 diabetes has gone up *700 percent.*[14] The standard American diet is likely to blame and the sad news is that a majority of these cases are preventable. Most people don't fully understand the devastating consequences of diabetes and even prediabetes, in which blood sugar levels are higher than normal but not yet high enough to qualify for a diagnosis of diabetes. High blood sugar levels damage blood vessels, inhibit healing, and damage every organ in the body. We have both lost loved ones with diabetes who had limbs amputated and suffered from depression, dementia, heart disease, and blindness.

Obesity is a serious national crisis with two-thirds of Americans overweight and one-third obese. Obesity increases inflammation, which is a low-level fire in the body that destroys our organs and is a risk factor for more than thirty medical illnesses, including cancer, diabetes, depression, and dementia. There are many published studies, including two by the research team at Amen Clinics, that report as your weight goes up, the size and function of your brain go down. This is the biggest brain drain in U.S. history and is now a national security crisis. Around 75 percent of young applicants for the military are rejected. The Department of Defense stated, "Being overweight or obese turns out to be the leading medical reason why applicants fail to qualify for military service. Today, otherwise excellent recruit prospects, some of them with generations of sterling military service in their family history, are being turned away because they are just too overweight."

Our national weight problem is not just an adult issue. Childhood obesity has increased from 4 percent in 1982 to 18.5 percent in 2015, a 350 percent increase. And it is very clear that the food scientists and fast-food companies are going after your kids. If you are not a warrior for the health of your brain and the brains of those who depend on you, ADD, depression, dementia, premature aging, diabetes, obesity, and premature death are the consequences for your loved ones and yourself.

When we first came to understand the interrelatedness of these illnesses and implemented integrated treatment strategies, we were so excited with the outcome for our patients: better energy, focus, mood, memory, weight, and even pain relief.

Initially, when we started to talk about the Brain Warrior's Way, some people pushed back, saying, "But I don't want to fight—being a Brain

The answer to these epidemic problems is not to see them as separate disorders with their own unique treatments, but rather as different expressions of the same unhealthy lifestyle that have exactly the same cure.
In other words, there are many ways to become sick, but there is one clear path to wellness, and it's simpler than you think:
It is the Brain Warrior's Way.

Warrior sounds hard." Our response was and still is, "Being sick is hard. Being a Brain Warrior is easy once you understand and implement the principles." Having your health, with better energy, memory, mood, and focus, is priceless. More than anything, being a Brain Warrior is an incredible mind shift with lifelong benefits—and you will never want to go back to bad habits and poor choices for your health.

We recently gave a presentation to the eighteen-member executive team of a multibillion-dollar technology company. At the end of the first morning, the CEO pulled Daniel aside and said he had to plant brain health in his company. "It could be our competitive advantage," he said, "especially when we are competing for talent with the likes of Google, IBM, and Microsoft." Just as it is for them, brain health is your competitive advantage in life. It will help you thrive in every aspect of your personal life, health, work, finances, and relationships.

■

There is a proverb in martial arts,
"Master, why do you teach me to fight, but
speak of peace?"
The master replies,
"It is better to be a warrior in a garden,
than a gardener in a war."

■

If you are a lover or a healer and not a fighter, like Daniel, then harness the healing power by becoming a peaceful Brain Warrior. The most effective warriors in human history never picked up a physical weapon. Think of Jesus, Gandhi, Nelson Mandela, and Martin Luther King Jr., all of whom inspired massive numbers of people to work for just causes and changed history forever. Their fights were personal and principle centered and were won with their brains, not their brawn, which is exactly what we will show you how to do.

If you are a fighter like Tana, who has black belts in both Tae Kwon Do and Kenpo, this book will make perfect sense to you, too. Tana has been through a war with her health and never wants to go through it again. As her sensei Bob White says, "If you are prepared for the worst, you can expect the best." For her, martial arts is symbolic of overcoming barriers and never giving up.

DANIEL AND TANA'S BRAIN WARRIOR PATHS

The Brain Warrior's Way is deeply personal for both of us. We love our mission of creating and leading the Brain Warrior community of people who are serious about the health of their bodies and brains. Here is a brief summary of our individual journeys, so you can understand why this movement is important to us.

DANIEL'S BRAIN WARRIOR PATH

The warrior mind-set has been with me since 1972 when I enlisted in the U.S. Army at the age of eighteen to become an infantry medic. Working with wounded soldiers was where my love of medicine was born. As a medic, I was a warrior servant and loved supporting the health of our fighting men and women. After about a year, I realized that as much as I loved the medical aspects of being a medic I really hated sleeping in the mud and being shot at, so I got myself retrained as an X-ray technician and developed a passion for medical imaging. As our professors used to say, "How do you know unless you look?"

In 1979, when I was a second-year medical student, someone I cared about deeply tried to kill herself, and I took her to see a wonderful psychiatrist. I came to realize that if he helped her, which he did, it would not only save her life, but it could also help her children, and even her future grandchildren, as they would be shaped by someone who was happier and more stable. I fell in love with psychiatry because I realized it has the potential to change generations of people.

Since deciding to become a psychiatrist, I have been at war nearly every day fighting for the mental health and brain health of my patients. I fight with them for their sanity, marriages, children, grandchildren, and jobs as well as their will to survive and thrive. In my work, I have been at war taking care of children, teenagers, and adults who have been suicidal, homicidal, scarred by trauma, psychotic, depressed, manic, panicked, addicted, and demented.

The journey to becoming a dedicated Brain Warrior began in earnest in 1991 when I attended my first lecture on brain SPECT imaging. SPECT stands for single photon emission computed tomography, a nuclear medicine study that looks at blood flow and activity in three-dimensional maps. SPECT was presented as a tool that could give psychiatrists more information to help their patients. In that one lecture, my two professional loves, medical imaging and psychiatry, came together and, quite honestly, revolutionized my life. Over the next twenty-five years my colleagues and I at Amen Clinics would build the world's largest database of brain scans related to behavior, totaling more than 125,000 scans of patients from 111 countries.

SPECT basically tells us three things about brain function: good activity, too little activity, and too much activity. Below are scans of people with traumatic brain injury and drug abuse. The images taught us many important lessons we will share with you in this book, such as how playing football, drinking too much alcohol, and using illicit drugs damage your brain and your life.

You've heard it said that a picture is worth a thousand words, but a map is worth a thousand pictures. A map tells you where you are and gives you directions on how to get to where you want to go. That is what SPECT imaging does for us at Amen Clinics. It gives us a map to help us better diagnose and treat our patients.

One of the first lessons the scans taught me was that "brain envy" is the real secret to happiness and longevity. When I first started to order scans I was so excited about the technology, I scanned many people I

TRAUMATIC BRAIN INJURY AND DRUG ABUSE

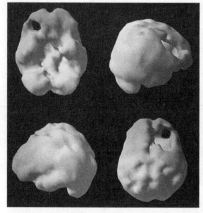 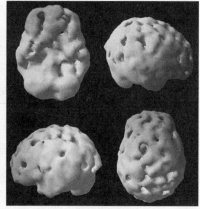

Low activity in the right frontal lobe from a traumatic brain injury

Holes indicate overall low activity, consistent with toxic effects of addiction

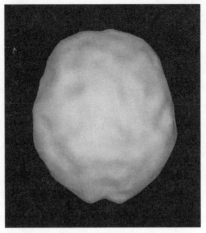

Full, even, symmetrical, healthy
appearance

knew, from a friend who had bad temper problems, to a cousin with a panic disorder, to my sixty-year-old mother, who happened to have a stunningly beautiful brain, which reflected her loving, amazing life.

I was thirty-seven the first time I was scanned, and my brain was not healthy. I played football in high school, contracted meningitis as a young soldier, and had many bad brain habits. I didn't sleep much, was chronically stressed, and carried an extra thirty pounds. Seeing my brain caused me to develop brain envy and really care about it. Besides, how could my sixty-year-old mother have a younger-looking brain than I did? That was really irritating. The Brain Warrior's Way program we are going to give you in this book is the same one I initially developed for myself and for our patients. Now, twenty-five years later, my brain looks younger and healthier, which is not usually what happens as we get older. Typically, brains become less and less active over time, but now we know it doesn't have to be that way. We've discovered that with the right strategies brain aging is optional.

■

The health of your brain is much more about
your actions than your age.

■

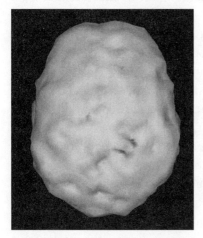 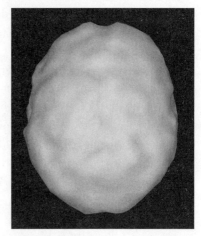

Bumpy, toxic appearance   Much healthier

TANA'S BRAIN WARRIOR PATH: YOUR HISTORY IS NOT YOUR DESTINY

The word *victim* conjures different emotions for everyone. I find it repulsive. It's personal. People who know me often describe me as an "ass kicker." It's true. I'm an ass kicker, a loving ass kicker, but an ass kicker nonetheless. My ass-kicking abilities were born of necessity. It would be fair to say I *did not* grow up in the All-American-Dream situation. In fact, reality television had nothing on my family. I was a little girl who grew up with a lot of trauma and drama. I still remember the day when I was four years old and saw my mother and grandmother falling to the floor sobbing in grief when they discovered that my uncle had been murdered in a drug deal gone wrong.

We were poor, so as a latch-key kid I soothed my anxiety with my best friends: the leprechaun (Lucky Charms), the captain (Cap'n Crunch), and the tiger (Frosted Flakes). The chronic stress in my house paired with the poor-quality food attacked my immune system. I was sick a lot and became a frequent flyer at the hospital. I earned my miles the hard way, but being in the hospital so frequently gave me the desire to help others who were sick.

When I was seven years old, my grandmother came to live with us because her diabetes had become unmanageable. It wasn't so that she could take care of me, but rather so I could help take care of her. By the time I was eleven, I had to inject her with insulin, because she had gone legally blind from the diabetes. My mother wasn't home to do it because she was working several jobs to make ends meet. I was terrified when the teaching nurse gave me an orange to practice on, telling me that if I gave my grandmother the wrong dose I could kill her.

The decision to learn how to fight, really fight, stems from a very personal traumatic experience. One day while walking to school at age fifteen, I was attacked by a large man. He clawed and grabbed very personal parts of my body as he overpowered me, pushing me toward the bushes in the nearby alley. Oddly, it didn't occur to me to be scared at the time, which ultimately may have saved my life. This psychopath in a suit was planning on raping me. Righteous indignation and fury were the only emotions coursing through my veins and gave me the fuel to scream, rip his shirt, slam my knee into his groin, and run . . . *fast*! Being overpowered is not a feeling you ever forget. Following the shock of that event, I felt terrified that any man could overpower me, simply because he was larger or stronger. Outrage quickly triumphed over terror. It took about a week before I resolved *never* to be a victim, or at least never act and feel like one. I taped a picture of Ms. Olympia to my mirror and began training to be strong, muscular, and agile. I wanted nothing to do with the image society was shoving down the throats of young women to be impossibly thin. I wanted to be a *warrior*!

What I never anticipated was the attack that came quietly eight years later, with no fanfare. Without warning a different kind of perpetrator knocked me flat on my back. It was a sucker punch I never saw coming. In fact it came from inside my own cells. I felt totally betrayed by my body when I was diagnosed with thyroid cancer in my early twenties. It had metastasized into my lymph nodes and recurred multiple times. For the next eleven years, while my friends were graduating from college and getting married, I was undergoing surgeries and radiation treatments and was dealing with a multitude of other health issues that followed as a result. For the second time I knew what it felt like to be a victim and I *despised* it. I became so depressed I literally prayed that I would die. I thought, "If there is a God, He has given up on me."

At one point I was so sick I was on nine prescriptions and taking medications just to handle the side effects of some of the drugs. When I complained, the doctor told me it was genetic, that I was in denial, and said maybe I should see a psychiatrist! Let me be clear: that is *not* how I met Daniel! I was never a patient at the clinics, even though Daniel often says I'm a psychiatrist's dream.

When I was sick, I was fighting an invisible phantom, and I realized I was in for the fight of my life. It was *so much harder* to fight for my own health. I was never given explanations about how I would respond physically and emotionally to the medical treatments I was undergoing. No one explained that when my thyroid gland was removed and I was taken off of thyroid medication for two months to go through treatments, I would feel so horrible that I would wish I were dead. The depression enveloped me like a dark cloud, and I couldn't see the sun to save my life. All I knew was that I couldn't get out of bed, and I would rather be dead than go on wasting oxygen and being a burden to my family. That's when I became certain that God had abandoned me.

But God hadn't given up on me. Somehow, over time, I managed to summon every ounce of power in my being and, with God's help, I transformed my anger and fear into a positive energy that fueled a phoenix-like rise from the ashes of poor health. I went on to become a different kind of warrior. That's when I became my own best health advocate.

What does growing up in poverty, having chronic stress, and being assaulted have to do with being attacked by cancer? A lot; chronic stress attacked my immune system and made me vulnerable to illness. I had to fight back, which is how I found my Brain Warrior path and decided to help myself and others transform their brains and bodies. I became a trauma/neurosurgical ICU nurse, and I took care of the sickest patients in the hospital. I also became a martial artist because it made me feel empowered and gave me the mind-set of a warrior.

The wisdom I gleaned from martial arts was more than fighting, more than a sport, more than an art. Being a warrior is a *mind-set.* Being a Brain Warrior is putting these concepts into a brain health model. *Anyone* can have a Brain Warrior mind-set with a little training and a lot of focus. I want to be an example of strength, health, and fitness for my daughter and my patients. I quickly realized that my martial arts training and my warrior mind-set combined to form the perfect metaphor to help empower patients who have felt weak, depressed, sick, and victimized. My goal is to teach you the way of the Brain Warrior so you can get a black belt in health.

FAST-TRACK VERSUS INCREMENTAL APPROACH

In our experience, there are two major types of people seeking help:

1. Some are like Tana and have a natural warrior mind-set. They want to jump in with both feet to feel better as quickly as possible. They are the kind of people who say, "Just tell me what to do and I'll do it all." They are often sick or they have experienced a major health crisis. They are tired of feeling sick and tired.

2. Other people will take an incremental approach. They will do one thing at a time, then another, then another, and over time plant as many good habits into their life that seem to make sense and are easily doable. This is more consistent with Daniel's path over the years.

Whichever path you choose, this program can help you. One of our most inspiring Brain Warriors, Nancy (whom you'll meet in Part 4), took the incremental approach and within a year lost 70 pounds and completely transformed her life. Daniel's father (you'll meet him in Part 7), on the other hand, was very sick, and when he jumped in to become a Brain Warrior he did everything we told him to, including changing his diet, exercising regularly, managing his stress, and taking his vitamins and supplements, and he powerfully transformed his health in a much shorter period of time. It is up to you to choose the path that is best for you; either one can lead you to great success.

BRAIN WARRIORS ADVANCE IN STAGES: PRIMITIVE, MECHANICAL, SPONTANEOUS

Every martial artist, athlete, or musician remembers how awkward she felt when she first started learning complex moves. Most felt like their bodies would never cooperate. However, over time the moves became smoother, until they eventually felt like second nature. The brain and body needed time to grow, make new connections, and adapt to new ways of working and thinking.

When someone is first starting the Brain Warrior's Way program she often feels a bit overwhelmed and confused.

- Hey, where's the sugar?!
- Everything in moderation!

- What happened to the bread and pasta? When are they coming back?
- But I love french fries and sodas!
- I don't know where to shop or what to buy!
- I don't want to get 8 hours of sleep!
- I don't want to exercise!
- I'm too busy, too stressed, too used to my old ways.

We tell our Brain Warriors in training not to worry, because they are in the **primitive phase,** when things feel impossible and hard, and they think they'll never be able to do it. It just takes trust, a bit of knowledge, success in feeling better quickly, and persistence to get to the next stage. Pretty soon, often within thirty days if you are on the fast track or thirty to ninety days if you are taking a more incremental approach, your taste buds regenerate themselves, the brain makes new connections and begins to grow, and soon enough, everything becomes easier.

Then you will transition to the **mechanical phase,** when you develop a healthy rhythm. You find the foods you love, exercises you can do, and brain healthy habits come easier to you. Clarity and energy replace brain fog. You start associating certain foods with feeling happier and more energized or with feeling sadder and more lethargic. It starts to become much easier to make healthy choices. You become better at noticing your negative thought patterns and begin questioning the negative thoughts running through your head. In this phase you still have to closely follow the Brain Warrior's Way program, because it is not yet second nature to you. This phase may last for one to three months for the fast-track folks and three to six months for the incrementalists.

Our goal is for you to reach the **spontaneous phase,** when your habits and responses become automatic and second nature. This usually occurs between four and six months for the fast-track folks and six and twelve months for the people who are taking things step by step. And if you persist through your challenges and setbacks, such as job or work challenges, divorce and deaths (which we all experience), the Brain Warrior's Way will last a lifetime.

In the spontaneous phase, the responses and habits become automatic.

- Do you want dessert? Yes, but I want something that serves my health, rather than steals from it.

- Do you want bread before dinner? No.
- Would you like a second glass of wine? No.
- You schedule your workouts and rarely miss them, as you would rarely miss your child's sporting event or a doctor's appointment. They are important to you.
- You don't have to think about your responses because they are spontaneous and habitual in a good way.

Get your black belt in brain health. Being a black belt doesn't mean you are tougher or stronger or that you don't get scared. Being a black belt means you never give up, you face your fears, you persevere, and you *always* get up one more time!

■

A black belt is just a white belt
who never quit.

■

This gives you permission to fall without failing, as long as you get up and try again. It is a process. Most important, you pass on the information by becoming a mentor to someone who is struggling. To get your black belt you are expected to be a mentor, to teach others your art. By teaching others, you powerfully reinforce in yourself what you've learned. It truly is in the giving that we receive.

PRIMITIVE—MECHANICAL—SPONTANEOUS

Based on our experience, the most successful Brain Warriors go through the following three phases over the course of a year.

Months One to Three: The Primitive Phase

In the primitive phase, just follow the steps and do what we ask you to do; it won't feel natural, so it is important to follow the map or you will get lost.

- Recognize the war for your health and make a decision to change (Mind-Set, Part 1)
- Assess your brain to know your type and get your important health numbers (Assess, Part 2)
- Clean out your pantry, stock your kitchen with great food, start some simple supplements (Sustenance, Part 3)
- Start developing brain healthy routines around exercise and sleep (Training, Part 4)
- Begin to identify your essence, and ask yourself why you really want to be healthy and clarify your purpose (Essence, Part 5)
- Think about who needs you to be healthy and who you are responsible for now and in the future, and look for friends who can do the program with you (Responsibility, Part 6)
- Don't think of this as a quick fix; complete the 14-Day Brain Boost (Yearlong, Part 7)
- Plan on making many mistakes; expect it, but don't think of falling as failing. To move to the mechanical phase, it is essential to pay attention to mistakes and start learning from them.

Months Two to Six: The Mechanical Phase

The mechanical phase is when your confidence begins to grow. You have the sense you can do it, but you still need a mentor and help.

- Become more committed to being a Brain Warrior sheepdog for yourself and loved ones, after becoming aware of the toxicity and illness around you. You are focused on the abundance of health rather than being deprived of treats. Increased success leads to increased determination. You are better at ignoring or deflecting the criticism of others; it is bound to come from your unhealthy friends. (Mind-Set, Part 1)
- Know the lab values of your important health numbers and work to optimize them. You attack vulnerability to disease on multiple fronts (inflammation, blood sugar control, antioxidant support, nutrient loading). You know your risk factors of depression, accelerated aging, and Alzheimer's and are actively taking steps to prevent them. (Assess, Part 2)

(CONTINUED)

- Find multiple foods you love that also love you back. Your supplements are more targeted to your brain type. (Sustenance, Part 3)
- Expand your brain healthy routines to include simple meditation, deep relaxation, and learning to question the negative thoughts that try to steal your happiness. You feel a continual need to keep learning. Your routine becomes easier and more defined. (Training, Part 4)
- Start to discuss your past failures and painful moments with friends and family and see the meaning in prior suffering. (Essence, Part 5)
- Start to share this message with friends, coworkers, and loved ones. Your Brain Warrior tribe becomes a critical part of your life. (Responsibility, Part 6)
- Feel all in, not for a few months, but for the rest of your life. (Yearlong, Part 7)
- Begin to make fewer mistakes. There will still be bad days, but you are better at learning from them and quickly turning them around.

Months Six to Twelve: The Spontaneous Phase

Habits become routine in the spontaneous phase. You say to yourself, "I got this; it is not hard." You naturally respond by doing the right things.

- Never think of giving up, even when you fall. You jump back into the game and start doing the right things again. You develop a sheepdog attitude and identify with being healthy. (Mind-Set, Part 1)
- Retest your important numbers to see your improvement. You're more focused on long-term prevention strategies. (Assess, Part 2)
- Find new foods and recipes, as if on a treasure hunt. Your nutrition and supplement routine is consistent. You feel joyful in your food choices and realize eating poorly is depriving yourself of your health. (Sustenance, Part 3)
- Feel uncomfortable or irritated when you are out of your Brain Warrior routine—it feels better to do the right thing than to do

the wrong thing. New learning excites you as you feel more focused and cognitively sharper. (Training, Part 4)

- Be excited to help others; being healthy and sharing the Brain Warrior message becomes part of who you are because you have a secret that can change the world. (Essence, Part 5)
- Become motivated to mentor others, to share your success. (Responsibility, Part 6)
- Celebrate the process of becoming a Brain Warrior and feeling better and stronger for a lifetime. (Yearlong, Part 7)

IS THIS PROGRAM FOR YOU?

This program is for those who want to be serious about their health, either out of desire or necessity. It is for people who want to look and feel their best for as long as possible and for those who want to excel at work and school and in their relationships. It is also for people who struggle with problems such as:

Depression
ADHD
Anxiety disorders
Post-traumatic stress disorder
Addictions
Bipolar disorder
Traumatic brain injuries
Memory problems
Early dementia
Alzheimer's disease or other forms of dementia in their families
Obesity
Diabetes or prediabetes
Heart disease
Cancer
Cognitive effects of chemotherapy

The Brain Warrior's Way is also for the parents of children with disabilities and those taking care of elderly or impaired parents. It is for those who want to build a legacy of health, rather than leave a legacy of illness; it's for those who want to be empowered; and it's for those who feel as if they were in a war for their health.

The Brain Warrior's Way is not for everyone. It is for people who want to change their brains and bodies for the rest of their lives. It is not for those looking for a quick fix, or cheat days, or wanting to take the month of December off. It is not for those who say "everything in moderation." Arsenic, cocaine, or having affairs in moderation can be very problematic. We are also not looking for people who have to be perfect. That is often an excuse to fail. We expect you will make mistakes and you will fall, just like toddlers fall when learning to walk, but Brain Warriors learn from their mistakes and make fewer and fewer of them over time.

We are recruiting and training Brain Warriors—people who are serious about the health of their brains and bodies, and the brains and bodies of those they love. Once you develop brain envy, a deep abiding love for the most precious organ in your body, you have the opportunity to become a Brain Warrior and everything changes for the good. The Brain Warrior's Way is a war cry to rally our families, businesses, schools, communities, and tribes to finally get and stay healthy. Join us.

PART 1

Mind-Set of a Brain Warrior

The War Is Won or Lost Between Your Ears

Efforts and courage are not enough without purpose and direction.

—JOHN F. KENNEDY

ARE YOU A WOLF, A SHEEP, OR A SHEEPDOG?

In his book *On Combat*, Lieutenant Dave Grossman talks about people being in one of three categories on a bell-shaped curve: wolves, sheep, or sheepdogs. Most people fall into the category of being sheep. They don't want trouble, and they don't cause trouble. Sheep willingly follow the status quo. Unfortunately, they will also follow other sheep off a cliff in total oblivion. Wolves are a very small percentage of the population. Wolves are predatory and prey on sheep. Sheepdogs, like wolves, also make up a small percentage of the population. Like wolves, they are aggressive and willing to fight. However, the powerful motivation of sheepdogs is what differentiates them from predators. They are fiercely protective of their flock.

Wolves are a powerful minority.

- Wolves target and take advantage of the weak.
- Wolves look for sheep that are not paying attention. When you are not paying attention to your health you are vulnerable to predators.
- Wolves prey on sheep that are sick. The sick are not likely to put up much of a fight.
- Wolves stalk sheep that have been separated from the herd. Loneliness and social isolation are associated with early death.[15]
- Wolves avoid sheep guarded by sheepdogs, even though the wolves are often stronger than the sheepdogs. Wolves want to avoid a fight or the possibility of being hurt.[16]

Sheep are the majority of people on the curve.

- Sheep are best known for their strong flocking behavior.[17] They go with the herd and do what the majority of the other sheep do.
- Sheep follow. When one sheep moves, the rest of the flock tends to follow, even when it's a bad idea. In Turkey in 2005, a sheep jumped off a cliff to its death; then 1,500 others followed.[18] In China in 2014, a lead sheep was blown off a cliff; 58 sheep dutifully followed it to their deaths.[19]
- Sheep are docile and usually nonaggressive, so they are easily led.
- Sheep don't want to believe that tragedy can or will occur.
- Sheep live in denial and don't want to see problems.
- Sheep pretend that all is okay and the wolf will never come.
- Sheep have two speeds—graze and stampede (groupthink).
- Sheep are often annoyed by sheepdogs—they remind them that trouble may be nearby. If your kids are annoyed by your sheepdog behavior, consider it normal.

Sheepdogs are at the other end of the bell curve; they are also a minority.

- Sheepdogs are purpose driven to protect their flock. They live to make a difference.
- Sheepdogs need training to be effective.
- Sheepdogs are serious. It is not a seasonal job.
- Sheepdogs love their flock, even when the love is not returned.
- Sheepdogs will give their lives to protect their sheep.
- Sheepdogs have a major advantage. They can survive in a hostile environment, while sheep cannot. When sheep get attacked, they often give in to death. When sheepdogs are attacked they fight back and are much more likely to survive.

We don't think many of our readers are likely to be wolves, but we urgently want you to stop acting like sheep, going to your early death and following others off the cliff, and instead start acting like sheepdogs, who are purposeful, serious, and protective of themselves and those they love.

SHEEPDOG BRAIN WARRIOR
MAJOR LAURIE HEISELMAN

Laurie is one of the best examples of a sheepdog Brain Warrior. When we met Major Laurie Heiselman, she was the director of one of the Salvation Army's largest drug treatment centers, located in Anaheim, California. She followed Daniel's work for many years and became excited about brain health. The more she learned, the more she realized that she had to get her own health under control to be a good example and took Tana's classes at Amen Clinics. Laurie ended up losing 55 pounds and a litany of her own health challenges, such as rosacea and irritable bowel issues.

As she got better, her husband started to engage in better health habits, as did her children and grandchildren. One of our favorite pictures is of Laurie drinking a green drink with her five-year-old grandson. As Laurie and her family got healthy, she realized she interacted with hundreds of substance abusers and staff at the Salvation Army who also desperately needed brain health.

Despite fierce and persistent opposition from her supervisors, Laurie created a brain healthy treatment program with our help. At the time it was painful and frustrating for us to watch Laurie desperately try to change an unhealthy culture; but as she persisted, the results for the

SHEEPDOG BRAIN WARRIOR LAURIE BEFORE AND AFTER

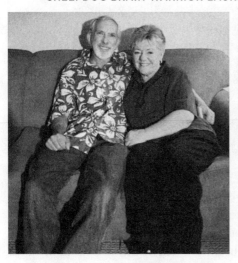
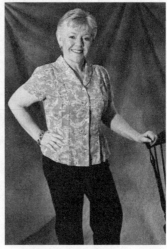

people under her care were truly spectacular. Many of the addicts showed improvement in moods, mental clarity, and judgment. There were fewer relapses and more success stories. Because Laurie was serious and became a Brain Warrior she not only felt better but created brain health in her family and in those she served.

BRAIN WARRIORS KNOW THEIR PURPOSE FOR BEING HEALTHY

The first principle of the Brain Warrior mind-set is to know your purpose, your why for getting and staying healthy. If you know your purpose at a deep emotional level you will refuse to be a sheep and you'll arm yourself with a sheepdog's attitude of being serious, guarding and fighting for your own life and the lives of those you love and serve. According to multiple studies, having a high sense of purpose is linked to decreased mortality from all causes.[20]

Two of the most important questions we ask our patients are

1. Why do you have to be healthy?
2. Why do you want a stronger mind and a more powerful brain?
   Is it to feel less anxious or less depressed?
   Is it to keep your mind healthy and enjoy your life for as long as possible?
   Is it to be able to stay connected to those you love?
   Who needs you to have a healthy brain?
   Who needs you to be their sheepdog?

■

If you don't know why you have to get healthy, you will never do the "what" of brain health.

■

Spend some time considering these two very important questions and write down, in as much detail as possible, your answers. Without understanding why you want to be healthy, it will be much more difficult for you to stay on track given the constant exposure to unhealthy choices in our culture.

We'd like to share our whys with you.

DANIEL: EMMY

Emmy, our five-year-old granddaughter, is my why for staying healthy. When she was only five months old, Emmy started to have wicked seizures. In one day she had 160 of them. I was lecturing in Boston when my daughter texted me videos of the seizures, in which it looked like Emmy was being electrocuted. Emmy was then diagnosed with a very rare genetic disorder associated with seizures, heart disease, and developmental delays. The neurologist told us she may never walk and had a 30 percent chance of dying before the age of three. He wanted to put her on a medicine that cost $26,000 a dose and was loaded with side effects, including wiping out her immune system.

I asked about trying the ketogenic diet, which has been found to be helpful for children with seizure disorders. Her doctor laughed at me and told me it didn't have any science supporting its use. Tana later told me she knew the relationship went sour when I asked the doctor if he knew how to read. "You're kidding me," I said. "It has over seventy studies showing it decreases seizure frequency by 50 percent in children, with some children becoming seizure free. The studies were done at a little place in Baltimore called Johns Hopkins. You've heard of Johns Hopkins?" I was furious.

The doctor said if we wanted to do the ketogenic diet he would not be Emmy's doctor. "You're fired," I replied. "How did you get through medical school without learning about informed consent? You're supposed to give us reasonable options and we decide what to do, remember?"

I then called the ketogenic clinic at Oregon Health & Science University and talked to their director, who told us the diet was an option for Emmy. Within three months of her going on the diet, her seizures went away, and by age three Emmy was walking to preschool. Now she is running. I am one of Emmy's sheepdogs.

I'm really clear on one of my major motivations for taking care of myself. I need to be healthy to fight for Emmy for as long as I can. If my brain is not healthy, I will never be my best for the people who need me. And if your brain is not healthy there is no way you can be your best for the people who need you. I never want to be a burden to my children. I want to be the leader of my family, but the only way that is possible is if I have a strong mind and a healthy brain. When I think of being tempted by ice cream or french fries versus keeping my brain healthy for Emmy, she always wins.

TANA: THREE WHYS

When I think about my purpose for getting and staying well, three are paramount.

1. I've been on the losing end of being sick and depressed. I'm never going down again without a fight. Being a Brain Warrior is symbolic of fighting for my health, empowerment, never giving up, and winning the war for my health!

2. Helping others become warriors for their brain and body is the mission God gave me. My healing process included becoming a mentor to others. I never imagined that I could turn the worst and even shameful experiences of my life into a message that empowers others. Pain shared is pain divided. Witnessing people heal on a daily basis is a blessing I'm not willing to waste.

■

Pain shared is pain divided.

■

3. I have a junior sheepdog to train and that's serious business. Your kids do what you do, not what you tell them to do. My daughter Chloe has my genes, which predisposes her to the same lousy health I've experienced. How she lives will determine whether she turns on health-promoting genes or disease-causing ones. I don't want her to experience the hell that I've gone through with my health. If I knowingly live an unhealthy lifestyle, she is likely to adopt my habits and be as sick as I was or worse. I'm Chloe's sheepdog, her protector, teacher, and role model.

Recently Chloe said, "Mom, why can't you be like the other moms in Newport Beach? Why can't you take me shopping and out for ice cream? You always take me and my friends to self-defense classes and health food places. You ate a sugar-free, gluten-free cupcake for my birthday. Why can't you just collect purses and go to lunch like normal moms? You always have bruises from training and you're so intense."

I said, "How you train is how you fight. If you don't train seriously, you will show up weak on fight day. How you live is how you'll respond when you have a health crisis or any other problem. You can't start training on fight day!" Then I asked if she wanted to trade me in.

Chloe rolled her eyes, paused, and said, "No, actually, it's pretty cool. I just don't always understand why you don't do things the easy way. You don't have to do all this. You could be at the mall and having lunch with your friends."

I hugged her and said, "Actually, most of my friends are warriors, not shoppers. Something tells me you will be much more intense than I am when you have little sheepdogs of your own to protect."

TANA AND CHLOE

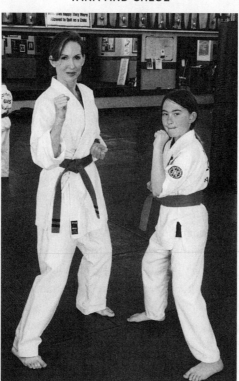

Even though there are times when Chloe pushes back against our healthy lifestyle, as most teens do, I'm always elated when I see our efforts pay off. Now and then we will get a call from a teacher or parent who relays how Chloe is proselytizing to her friends. She has been heard telling them, "You could be making better choices." She might not want us to know it's sinking in, and that's okay. It's how she shows up in life that matters.

We know Emmy and Chloe need us, but we also need them. Whatever your reasons for being healthy are, now is the time to start.

BRAIN WARRIORS IDENTIFY WITH BEING STRONG, SERIOUS, AND HEALTHY

The basic difference between an ordinary man and a warrior is that a warrior takes everything as a challenge, while an ordinary man takes everything as a blessing or a curse.

—CARLOS CASTANEDA, *THE WHEEL OF TIME*

When people begin the shift to identifying as a Brain Warrior, they start to think and behave differently. They become more serious about their health and understand the importance of making good decisions; they stop complaining about giving up the treats, they stop saying "everything in moderation," and they stop taking the month of December off from their health plan. This mind-set shift is one of the most critical aspects of success. Without it you are doomed to yoyo dieting and falling back forever.

"Everything in moderation" is the thought that's ruining your health.[21] If you listen to the people who say it, they are often unhealthy. It is an excuse to do the wrong things for your brain and body. It leads to thinking that alcohol is a health food, eating more sugar than you need, and sitting in front of the television for hours. Everyone defines *moderation* differently, but it is usually in favor of doing the things that hurt your health.

Understanding who you are and what you want in life is important for guiding your behavior and decisions. How would you answer these two questions:

1. Who do you desire to be? Create a personal mission statement for your life.

For Tana: "I am a living example of health, fitness and empowerment."
For Daniel: "The only way I am an effective messenger is if I live the message of my life."

2. What do you truly want in life?

We both desire health, energy, lasting cognitive function, contribution, creativity, passion, abundance, and fun.

What do *you* want? Write it down and look at it every day.

Write out five to eight positive reasons you have for wanting to become a Brain Warrior. For example:

1. I will have better energy.
2. I will have better focus.
3. I will have better memory.
4. I will have a better mood.
5. I will protect my brain now and in the future.
6. I will be a role model for those who need me.
7. I can rock my mission with passion and fun.
8. I can support my immune system so my cancer won't come back.

Write out five to eight pain points you want to avoid by becoming a Brain Warrior. For example:

1. I want to avoid hurting myself.
2. I want to avoid being sicker, sadder, and less cognitively aware.
3. I want to avoid damaging my brain.
4. I want to avoid being less effective in my life.
5. I want to avoid being a poor role model to those I love.
6. I want to avoid negatively affecting future generations by turning on the disease-promoting genes that I pass on.
7. I want to avoid the return of my cancer.
8. I want to avoid the financial burden that comes with being sick.

BUT HOW CAN I HAVE ANY FUN?

Some people have a difficult time thinking like a healthy person because they believe they can have fun only when they are doing things that are actually bad for them. For example, we have a high school course called Brain Thrive by 25 that is taught in forty-two states and seven countries. Whenever we teach the things students should avoid if they want a healthy brain, a smart-mouthed teenage boy will invariably blurt out, "But how can I have any fun?"

In fact, when we scanned famous basketball player Dennis Rodman during an episode of *Celebrity Rehab with Dr. Drew* and showed him his alcohol-damaged brain, he asked Daniel the same question.

So, whenever we get this question we play a game, with kids and adults alike, and ask,

> "Who has more fun? The person with the good brain or the one with the bad brain?"

Q: Who gets the girl and gets to keep her, because he doesn't act like a jerk . . . the guy with the good brain or the one with the bad brain?
A: The guy with the good brain.
Q: Who gets into the college they want to get into . . . the teen with the good brain or the one with the bad brain?
A: The teen with the good brain.
Q: Who gets the best jobs and keeps them . . . the woman with a good brain or the one with the bad brain?
A: The woman with the good brain.
Q: Who makes the most money . . . the person with the good brain or the one with the bad brain?
A: The person with the good brain.
Q: Who is the best parent . . . the dad with the good brain or the one with the bad brain?
A: The dad with the good brain.

Whatever it is you want in life, it is easier to achieve when your brain works right, but it starts with knowing why you care and shifting into identifying yourself as a Brain Warrior.

Before Tana tested for her second martial arts black belt in Kenpo, she was nervous and unsure of herself, despite having already earned a black belt in Tae Kwon Do. She was older and felt that the Kenpo black belts who would test her were tougher and better trained. It was not until she shifted her mind-set from "Someday I *may be* a black belt" to "I *am* a black belt, I am strong, I am a warrior," that she lost her anxiety and performed at a very high level. She developed her own phrases that motivated her, such as "No way, not today." She changed "I will be someday" to "I am now." To help you become a Brain Warrior, develop a powerful phrase for yourself or borrow one of ours.

■

Defeat is a state of mind.
No one is ever defeated until defeat has
been accepted as a reality.

■

BRAIN WARRIOR KYLE

Kyle, one of the people Tana looks up to, is a seventh degree black belt in martial arts and a retired undercover police officer. When we first started working with him he made the statement, "I just can't give up Pepsi and bread. It's too hard."

Tana laughed and said, "All the fighters I work with amaze me! It makes me want to laugh every time I hear one of you say something dumb like that. Let's see . . . getting a black belt is hard; getting a seventh degree black belt is *really hard*! Having a successful career as a competitive martial artist is hard! Being an undercover police officer is insanely hard and dangerous. . . . This is *not hard*—it's a mind-set. When you walk onto the mat, do you start by telling yourself, 'This is hard; I'm going to give up today?' When you walk into a drug bust with a bunch of gang-bangers, do you tell yourself you're going to lose? If not, why do you do it with Pepsi? Are you really willing to lose the most important fight of your life to a 12-ounce *can of Pepsi* or a fluffy baguette?"

Looking like a sheepish child, Kyle said, "Wow! I feel so silly. I never thought of it as though I were losing a fight to a can of soda, even though I'm on several medications and my doctor keeps telling me I have to give it up. If I look at it that way, I can do this." Kyle started the program and went on to lose 40 pounds over the following three months and felt happier and stronger than he had in many years.

BE A GOOD PARENT TO YOURSELF: FIRM AND KIND

We see people allowing their spoiled, bratty inner child get away with what they'd never allow from their children. So many of our patients stay stuck, singing the same old refrain, "I want what I want when I want it. I don't want to be deprived." They're seeking help for health problems, but when they're given the solution, they kick, whine, and cry. They want a magic pill instead of a logical solution. You need to start being a better parent to yourself.

As a child psychiatrist, Daniel says the best parents are those who are "firm" and "kind." Children need clear direction and clear lines of authority, and they need an atmosphere of love and kindness. You are the same way. We want you to treat yourself with love and kindness, but stop giving in to your inner child, who continually throws tantrums to get his or her way. Stop giving in to your own bad behavior! We were with a client recently who was struggling with his weight. He said he often felt as though he had to give in to his cravings. He had three teenage boys, and one of them had significant behavior problems that Daniel had treated. We asked him how his troubled son would be if he always gave in to his temper tantrums. Do you think he would get better or worse? "Worse, of course," he said. When you give in to your own tantrums you are creating your own internal behavior disorder, which is ruining your health and killing you early. Be a loving, effective parent to yourself. Don't give in when you know your inner child is being whiny and bratty and demanding unhealthy food or poor choices that put your health at risk.

BRAIN WARRIORS FOCUS ON ABUNDANCE, NEVER DEPRIVATION

When making dietary changes, many people give up because they focus on what they cannot have rather than what they can have, which is a deprivation mind-set. They focus on the loss of fast, pesticide-laden, sugary foods that drive inflammation and hijack their taste buds. Yet, when they actually eat high-quality food, they find that their taste buds come alive (it takes about ten days), and food tastes better than ever. Brain Warriors understand that getting well includes focusing on an abundance of the right things and depriving yourself of illnesses, such as diabetes, heart disease, cancer, depression, and dementia. Changing your focus is a critical shift.

During one scene in the movie *City Slickers*, Curly, a rough old cowboy (played by Jack Palance), is riding horses with Mitch (Billy Crystal), a city dweller who is trying to rediscover the meaning of his life. Curly says to Mitch, "Do you know what the secret to life is?" as he holds up the index finger of his right hand.

"Your finger?" Mitch replies with a quizzical look.

"One thing . . . just one thing," Curly replies in a deep voice. "You stick to that and everything else don't mean s—t."

"That's great, but what's the one thing?" asks Mitch.

"That's what you have to figure out," Curly replied.

A few scenes later Curly dies without ever telling Mitch what the one thing was. Mitch was beside himself, wanting to know what it was.

Getting well is never about deprivation. But it is about getting your priorities straight. Would you rather give in to temptation in the moment or choose your health and longevity? You have the power to make this choice multiple times a day.

Last year we were working with a patient named Mark, who struggled with ADD, depression, and his weight. He was having trouble sticking to the routine he knew was good for him. As we discussed his roadblocks to getting and staying well, he said something very profound.

"I don't want to deprive myself. That's how I feel. I want what I want when I want it."

"So what do you want most?" we asked. "Your health, a great brain, and years added to your life or the alcohol and sugar?"

"Of course I want brain health—that's why I'm here."

Then we told Mark about the one thing. "The one thing is that when you do the right thing you stop feeling deprived. You are getting stuck in a two-year-old's mind-set. You should feel deprived when you do the wrong thing because you are depriving yourself of what you really want most—good health, energy, a sharp memory, and the ability to control your life and manifest your purpose."

Getting well is about an abundance of the things that drive your health. Without the right mind-set, there are too many land mines in our society waiting to sabotage your success. Having an abundance mind-set is critical to getting and staying well.

BRAIN WARRIORS ARE ACCURATE, HONEST, AND CAUTIOUSLY OPTIMISTIC THINKERS

And you shall know the truth, and the truth shall set you free.

—JOHN 8:32

Here's something you won't read every day from health-care professionals: "Positive thinking kills way too many people." Two of the most dangerous mind-set weapons of mass destruction are *mass denial* and *having anxiety that is too low*.

Mass denial prevents people from doing anything significant about the health problems they face. Unfortunately, there is no other way to talk about it when 50 percent of Americans are prediabetic or diabetic and 67 percent are overweight or obese. We want you to know the truth about the health of your brain and body, and we want you to do something about it if you are headed for trouble or are in trouble already. That is why in Part 2 we'll tell you how critical it is to know your important health numbers, such as body mass index (BMI) and markers of inflammation. When you break through your denial you will be much more serious about your health and more willing to live the Brain Warrior's Way.

In regard to anxiety, having some is absolutely critical to good health and success. Levels of anxiety that are too low are associated with underestimating risks, a lackadaisical attitude toward your health, and making bad decisions. Imagine warriors who were not vigilant, even when the enemy was nearby. What would happen? Early defeat and death to them and their entire tribe would have been the likely result. The same principle applies to your health. One of the reasons we wrote this book is that we want you to be serious about your health, know the weapons, agents, and attitudes of mass destruction, and protect yourself and your loved ones as much as possible.

The way you think dramatically affects how you feel and every decision you make. The lies you tell yourself are one of the biggest factors that drive illness and early death. Here are some of the most common and destructive lies we hear.

"I don't want to deprive myself." Doesn't eating bad food deprive you of your health, your most precious resource? What is worth more? Energy, a trim waistline, and health or the mountain of fries, sodas, cakes, cookies, and the like you have consumed over the last decade?

"I can't eat nutritious foods because I travel." We are always amused by this one, because we travel a lot. It just takes a little forethought and planning.

BRAIN WARRIOR JASON

After coming to the clinic, Jason, a former Marine, was told that he needed to incorporate our lifestyle program for the best results in his treatment plan. Jason had a previous brain injury, had ADD, had trouble focusing, and was overweight. He complained to Tana that he couldn't get healthy because he traveled more than 200 days per year for work. It was hard. Tana, in her usual loving way, called him out. She asked, "Are you a baby or a Marine? I thought Marines were tough," and proceeded to tell him the only reason he couldn't do it was because he didn't care enough. She then gave him strategies that would help him when he was on the road. A few months later, Jason wrote her this letter.

Tana:

I love the way you throw it down. I'm on the road about 200 days/year and rarely in the same spot longer than 3 days. Like you said then, it's all in the preparation. I now make sure that every hotel room includes a refrigerator and that my itinerary includes directions from the rental car facility to a grocery store that is known to be open when I arrive.

My focus has been a lot better but even more noticeable has been my ability to have control over my food impulses and clarity of thought as a whole. For the first time since Marine Corps Boot Camp in 1999, I'm sleeping 7.5–8 hours every night. Just like everything else my sleep schedule is scheduled with purpose. I am working out. I call the day passes at the various gyms wherever I happen to be just part of the 6 pack tax (stolen from Tim Ferris). Point being is that there are no more excuses for not working out or eating healthy regardless of where I find myself.

As it stands now, I'm down about 35lbs since Thanksgiving (about 6 weeks) and the entire experience has been almost easy and definitely fun! Not too bad for a holiday season. . . . All areas of life seem to be opening up and I don't think my gratitude has ever been so high. . . . I'm getting my twenties body back and loving it.

Truth be told things are now easiest on the road . . . so much easier to plan for (because there is a strategy) than being at home even which is GREAT for me. :)

Words can't describe the peace that comes with finally understanding things a bit more. I can't thank you enough. Thank you!

Jason Stuber

Acknowledge the excuses and let them go. They're not serving your best interests and they're only crutches to prevent you from living your best life.

"My whole family is overweight; it is in my genes." This is one of the biggest lies. Genes account for only 20 to 30 percent of your health. The vast majority of health problems are driven by the bad decisions people make. Daniel's genetic test says he is likely to be fat, but he isn't because he stopped making the bad decisions that would have made it likely for him to be so.

"I can't afford to get healthy." Being sick is always more expensive than getting healthy. According to the Harvard School of Public Health eating healthful foods costs an extra $1.50 a day.[22] Over time, having a healthy brain and body will be worth so much more than that small amount of money.

"I can't find the time to work out." With a sharper mind, you will actually save time if you work out.

"It's Easter, Memorial Day, July Fourth, Labor Day, Thanksgiving, Christmas, Monday, Tuesday, Wednesday, Thursday, Friday, Saturday, or Sunday." There is always an excuse to hurt yourself. When you stop believing every stupid thought you have, the quality of your decisions and your health will go way up.

Here are more lies that drive failure:

"I'll start tomorrow." Tomorrow never comes. You will be better off starting today.

"They serve only bad food at work." Then bring your lunch to work.

"My memory is no good, but that is normal at my age." We actually hear this lie from people who are thirty-five, forty-five, fifty-five, sixty-five, and older. The truth is that most memory problems are not due to your age, but your bad habits.

We recently recorded an interview with Todd, a fifty-three-year-old high-level business executive who told us his memory was terrible. "I am sure it is just my age. I am just getting older," he said. "I often have no idea where I put my keys and sometimes find them in the refrigerator, next to the eggs."

"It is definitely not normal," we replied. "It is one of the little lies people tell themselves to justify their memory problems and bad habits. The denial prevents them from getting the help they need. Tell us about your diet and exercise."

When Todd heard mention of exercise he perked up. "I exercise five times a week. I run long distances and am in great shape."

Something wasn't making sense. "What about your diet?" we asked.

"Every morning I have a Diet Coke and Pop-Tarts in the car on the way to work. The rest of the day doesn't get much better."

One of Tana's eyebrows went up, in the funny way it does when she thinks, "Seriously?" Putting toxic fuel in a car will definitely decrease its performance. Putting toxic fuel in your body will definitely hurt your brain, no matter how much exercise you do.

"If you had a million-dollar racehorse," we asked, "would you ever give it junk food?"

"Of course not," he said.

"You are so much more valuable than a racehorse. It's time to treat yourself with a little love and respect," we encouraged.

Three months later, Todd told us his memory had significantly improved. He also said we haunt him at every meal. We are hoping to do the same for you.

We want you to always tell yourself the truth. Unwarranted positive thoughts can be as destructive as negative, hateful, hopeless, or helpless thoughts.

BRAIN WARRIORS ARE AWARE OF MASS PROPAGANDA AND WEAPONS OF PSYCHOLOGICAL WARFARE

Once you are a Brain Warrior and aware of the dangers in the environment, you will begin to notice all of the advertising directed to hook your brain. What do the following slogans have in common, besides the fact that they are still stuck in your brain decades after they were created?

"I'm loving it."

"Finger lickin' good."

"Have it your way."

"Open happiness."

"You deserve a break today."

"Oh I wish I was an Oscar Mayer wiener . . ."

"They're grrrrreat!"

"Silly rabbit, Trix are for kids!"

"They're magically delicious."

"Breakfast of champions."

"Melts in your mouth, not in your hand."

"Bet you can't eat just one."

These slogans were all designed to target your *children*. These foods, with their catchy jingles, were also created to win the "stomach share" of our tiny consumers by targeting the bliss point in their brains. Hold on, this gets really interesting, albeit very annoying.

In the 1970s a mathematician by the name of Howard Moskowitz discovered that the perfect combination of sugar, salt, and fat would optimize the human brain's pleasure experience. He coined it the "bliss point." Fast-forward a few decades, and we now know that triggering the bliss point not only increases sensory experiences like taste and texture but activates an area deep in the brain, called the nucleus accumbens, which is associated with motivation and pleasure. The nucleus accumbens is the same part of the brain that is activated by certain drugs such as cocaine, methamphetamines, nicotine, and morphine! In other words, the job of food designers is to create foods that hook your brain, just like addictive drugs. "Bet you can't eat just one!" They weren't kidding.

Moskowitz became a food engineering rock star, sought after by most major food manufacturers when the bliss point was discovered. In fact he became a game changer in the food industry, starting a war to win stomach share, similar to market share. The more stomach share that food companies control, the more real estate they dominate in grocery stores; and guess which shelves have the most market value. The lower one-third, the ones that have the foods your kids can reach. When your kids grab those sugary foods in colorful packages, they nag, scream, throw themselves on the floor, and hold on to them until you say yes. Turns out it's not totally their fault. Their bliss point has been triggered! Think of this as a long-term investment on the part of major food companies.

When questioned about his role in the increasing epidemic of childhood obesity and illness, Moskowitz had this to say: "There's no moral issue for me. I did the best science I could. I was struggling to survive and didn't have the luxury of being a moral creature." To some degree he's right. He was just the brain behind the mega-money machines bidding for his talent. And if it hadn't been him, eventually it would have been someone else, and eventually there *were* many others. There was simply too much money at stake for something as minor as *health* to get in the way of addictive food!

Lunchables, created as a way to sell more bologna, and marketed by Kraft, is one of the products of this race to trigger the bliss point. It is arguably one of the *least healthful* lunch products on the market for children, yet has sales near a billion dollars a year. Geoffrey Bible, former CEO of Philip Morris (which previously owned Kraft), was reported to have said that the most nutritious part of Lunchables is the napkin! He made it clear that there were no plans to change it when he said, "Well, that's what the consumer wants, and we're not putting a gun to their head to eat it. That's what they want. If we give them less, they'll buy less, and the competitor will get our market," according to a 2013 *New York Times Magazine* article.

Bob Drane, previous vice president of Oscar Mayer, was quoted in the same article as saying, "Our limbic brains love sugar, fat, salt . . . so formulate products to deliver these. Perhaps add low-cost ingredients to boost profit margins. Then 'supersize' to sell more, and advertise and promote to lock in 'heavy users.' Plenty of guilt to go around here!"

But Philip Morris isn't the only villain. The race was on to find new and creative ways to target the bliss point. Here are a few of the weapons they discovered.

- Vanishing caloric density or "meltness": Foods that melt quickly make the brain think there are fewer calories; hence you eat more.
- Sensory-specific satiety: Researchers discovered how to override the brain's signal for sensory satiety by not including *one distinct, overwhelming flavor* (this is why cooking with healthful spices helps you feel satisfied sooner).
- Perfect crunchiness: The perfect break point is 4 pounds of pressure.
- Texture: Removing fiber increases the ease of food sliding down the throat as well as the pleasure sensation. Fiberless food also means you can eat your food faster and get out of the fast-food restaurant in less time, meaning they can serve more bodies in a single day.
- Aroma: Flavor is enhanced by aroma. In fact, humans only have five major taste sensations (sweet, sour, bitter, salty, and umami—savory, as in meat broth or tomato sauce). Other nuances are created through smell. That's why Cinnabon places ovens at the front of the store and has a schedule to bake fresh rolls every 30 minutes. Between times they often bake brown sugar and cinnamon just to create the enticing aroma that patrons seem helpless to resist.

Yet, society and corporations blame you for being overweight or sick because you lack self-control, portion control, or inadequate exercise. We wonder how you can have self-control when the food scientists have been using sophisticated neuroscience and plotting against your brain for decades.

These companies are after our kids and we are fighting back! If anyone is going to bribe or brainwash our kids, it's going to be us! That's why we have Junior Brain Warriors in training. We began playing games with our daughter and grandkids to teach them about healthful eating. If anyone is going to give our kids toys for eating food, it's going to be us—and it's going to be for eating nutritious foods. We create scavenger hunts, treats, games, and fun meals as a way to get them excited about nutrition and brain health. Get your kids and grandkids started in Junior Brain Warrior training now!

BRAIN WARRIORS ARE AWARE TROUBLE POTENTIALLY LURKS IN HOSPITALS, DOCTORS' OFFICES, SCHOOLS, BUSINESSES AND CHURCHES

Not only are the media constantly blasting unhealthy messages to you, but when you open your eyes and observe with a Brain Warrior mind-set, you will see that there are sick choices all around you. When you become aware of all the potential land mines it shifts everything; you will be more thoughtful, and this will lead you to make better choices. Know better, do better.

Until recently, the Cleveland Clinic, a hospital known for its "innovative technology," had one of the world's busiest-per-square-foot McDonald's on its premises. Does this strike you as an obvious conflict of interest? About eight years ago we went to an appointment for Tana to see a new endocrinologist. He had bowls of candy and cookies in the waiting room. Ironically, sick people can go to the doctor, or a well-known medical clinic, and freely snack on food that makes them sicker. Unbelievable! Over the last decade as our work has focused more on the connection between physical and emotional health, we have realized that many schools, businesses, hospitals, and churches could do a much better job of helping the people they serve.

On a Sunday morning in August 2010 we went to a church near our home and Daniel told Tana that he would save them seats while Tana dropped Chloe off at children's church. As Daniel walked toward the sanctuary he passed hundreds of doughnuts for sale for charity, which really irritated him, even though he had seen doughnuts at church ever since he was three years old. Then he walked by bacon and sausage cooking on the grill, and his irritation escalated. And then, just before he walked into the sanctuary, he passed hundreds of hot dogs being grilled for after-church fellowship. He felt the heat rising in his neck. Then as he sat down, he heard the minster talking about the ice cream festival they'd had the night before.

Daniel was so frustrated that when Tana found him in church he was typing on his phone, which Tana absolutely hates; she gave him the look—the one only a wife can give—that said, "Why are you on that thing in church!? Don't you know you are going to hell?" Then Daniel showed her what he was writing:

```
Go to church . . . get doughnuts . . .
bacon . . . sausage . . . hot dogs . . .
ice cream. They have no idea they are
sending people to heaven EARLY! Save them,
then kill them. This is not the plan!
```

When we open our eyes and become aware, we see evidence that our society, including our public schools, churches, and doctors' waiting rooms, however well meaning, are hurting us with the food they offer. There is a better way, and we have to do more to improve the food choices in our environment. **Food pollution is killing us.** During that service Daniel prayed that God would use us to help change the food at places of worship. The House of God, no matter what religion, should not be a place that promotes illness.

Two weeks later Pastor Rick Warren called Daniel. Rick is the senior pastor at Saddleback Church, one of the largest churches in America. He is also the author of *The Purpose-Driven Life,* which has sold over 35 million copies worldwide. Rick told Daniel, "Last Sunday I baptized about 800 people. About halfway through I realized everyone was fat. Then I realized I was fat and a terrible example to my congregation. Will you help us?"

With his prayer still fresh in his mind, Daniel said, "You had me from hello." Together with Rick and our friend Dr. Mark Hyman, we created the Daniel Plan, a five-step program to get the world healthy through churches. The first week 15,000 people signed up for the program. Within the first year they lost *more than 250,000 pounds.* The plan is now being done in thousands of churches worldwide.

Being aware is one of the first critical steps to truly getting healthy, and when you are aware, you will quickly realize you are in a war that can be won by becoming a Brain Warrior.

Whenever we are on the Saddleback Campus we hear story after story of how lives have been changed, using the principles outlined in this book. People have told us:

- "I've lost 20 . . . 30 . . . 40 . . . 90 . . . 150 pounds"
- "My numbers are so much better!"
  - ► Cholesterol was 202, now 164
  - ► Blood pressure was 142/92, now 125/75
  - ► BMI was 35.7, now 26.1

- "No more headaches! It's amazing. I was taking prescription pain medication almost daily. It's been more than two weeks without any pain or pills!"
- "My clothes fit loosely and I can get back into my old ones."
- "Color is coming back to my gray hair . . . who knew?"
- "My mood is so much more stable and positive."
- "My asthma is better."
- "With the elimination of sugar, flour, salt, and processed foods, I rarely have any cravings and have found I eat smaller amounts of nutrient-rich foods."
- "I just finished chemo. Everyone is amazed at how much energy I have and how fast my hair is returning. I am running circles around a friend who is ten years younger and doesn't have cancer. (He is not on the plan.)"
- "My complexion looks great; the improvement in the smoothness of my skin is remarkable."
- "Ninety-eight percent of my headaches at night have disappeared. I wake up feeling clearheaded instead of foggy."
- "I don't have body, joint, or muscle pain in the mornings."
- "I'm off my high blood pressure meds . . . and am working on getting off of my type 2 diabetes and cholesterol meds."
- "I am diabetic. Now my blood sugar is dramatically better than when I was on insulin. I am not on it anymore."
- "I'm having less arthritis (inflammatory) pain."
- "Odd to say this in church, but my sex life has dramatically improved!"

We have heard many, many stories of transformation from the thousands of people who have shifted to the Brain Warrior's mind-set. Not only do they inspire others but they also inspire us to continue doing the work we are so passionate about. Angie's story is one of the ones that really touched our hearts:

BRAIN WARRIOR ANGIE

Dear Daniel and Tana,

My story starts when I was very young. I mostly ate TV dinners, except when my very Italian grandmother loved me with food. By age 8 I felt "fat" and was sent to Jenny Craig (at age eight!). My mom was very concerned about my appearance. I was already experiencing the nag of food addiction and felt like there was something wrong with me. I would hide in the kitchen closet binging. I always had a poor body image even though my weight was "ok" because I was active. I continued searching for my mom's approval, who I always felt was watching me with disapproval. As a result, I would buy mass amounts of garbage food and hide by myself, binging on it. The pain and shame were unbearable.

It wasn't until I found your program that I successfully let go of the food addiction! What a revelation to realize that the food I was eating was the problem and not me! It was like the heavens opened up!

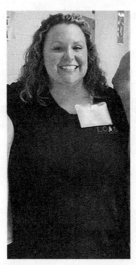 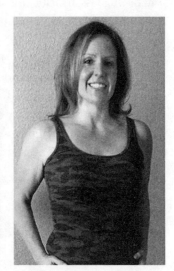

Before   After

I was very young when I got married and had a baby. Having no idea how to take care of a family, we ate garbage for nearly a decade. However, I tried every diet, pill, and quick fix I researched—only to fail again and again. We bought into the low-fat diet crap, which led me to become 225 pounds at 5 feet tall.

My marriage wasn't happy. How could it be? When my husband started losing weight with portion control it only made me more unhappy. He tried helping me, which only made me angry, like an addict defending my addiction. But I was worried too, so why couldn't I stop eating?

It all changed in May 2014 when a coworker recommended your program and mentioned Tana's name after visiting Amen Clinics. I thought to myself that it was just another program I would fail, but got the program anyway. When I started reading I felt hope, real hope! I read it from cover to cover within a few days. Imagine: my anxiety and depression could be a result of my poor diet? I had tried gluten-free programs before, but never controlled my cravings.

This program was so different! You promised a change in two weeks. Boy, were you right! I lost eleven pounds in the first two weeks. I've lost 103 pounds total. I weigh 122 pounds! I went from a size 18/20 to a size 3/4. I live and love to eat healthy and exercise! I never miss junk food and I can find something healthy to eat anywhere I go, or I pack a bag of food. I've learned so much!

My confidence is so high, and people notice. I receive so many compliments on my appearance. I no longer avoid social activities or feel like people are ridiculing me. Your program inspired me to take control of my own health and now I have the tools to do it! I took what I learned and applied it to daily life and now I am inspiring others to lose weight too. If I can do this program, anyone can!

I can't say I have gotten MY old life back, this is better than any place I have ever been! This has been an emotional journey filled with much pain and sickness, which has now been released. My life is changing in amazing ways. I feel daily gratitude and confidence in myself!

Before:

> *Migraine headaches*
> *Rosacea*

Dry skin
Dizziness
Stomach problems
Brain fog
Ovarian cysts
Anxiety and depression that ruled my life

After:

Lost 103 pounds in 14 months
Present for my family
No digestive issues or cysts
Empowered
Highest confidence ever
Clear mind—No migraines
Control over moods
STRONG NOT SICK
Able to forgive more easily
Dramatic improvement in focus
I am stronger than my anxiety and Depression!
Even though I don't know how to cook I'm able to do it!

It wasn't hard to do over the holidays once I knew what to do and had lost my cravings. I made several dishes and took them with me to gatherings. My family became curious and supportive. If I can do this, anyone can do this! Your program has helped me in so many ways. Tana's story inspired me and this program helped me gain control of my life. I am forever grateful. I give your book as a gift to my friends now, with the hope that they will go where I have gone.

Love and gratitude!
Angie

Brain Warrior Mind-Set Takeaways

Check those that apply to you:

- ❏ I am a Brain Warrior sheepdog.
- ❏ I know my purpose for being healthy.
- ❏ I identify with being strong, serious, and healthy.
- ❏ I focus on abundance, never deprivation.
- ❏ I know the one thing.
- ❏ I am an accurate, honest, cautiously optimistic thinker.
- ❏ I am aware of the mass-propaganda weapons and psychological warfare.
- ❏ I am aware that trouble lurks even in hospitals, doctors' offices, schools, businesses, and churches.

We encourage you to work on any of these statements that you did not check. The statements you did not check are areas for you to potentially work on.

PART 2

Assessment of a Brain Warrior

Getting Ready to Win the War

The supreme art of war is to subdue the
enemy without fighting.

—SUN TZU

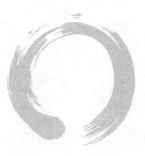

THE NUMBER ONE STRATEGY FOR HEALTH, SUCCESS, AND LONGEVITY

In 1921, American psychologist Lewis Terman initiated a longitudinal study on 1,548 gifted ten-year-old children. Terman and, after his death, other researchers followed these individuals for the next eighty years, looking for traits associated with success, health, and longevity. Howard Friedman and Leslie Martin published an update of the results of this research in their book, *The Longevity Project: Surprising Discoveries for Health and Long Life from the Landmark Eight-Decade Study.*[23] What was the surprise? The secret to living a long life had nothing to do with happiness, a lack of stress, avoiding hard work, or a lack of worry. In fact, the don't-worry-be-happy people died the earliest from accidents and preventable illnesses. The secret was living conscientiously and using forethought, planning, and perseverance in all aspects of one's life. Conscientiousness was the number one predictor of longevity.

Friedman and Martin offered a number of reasons conscientious people stay healthier longer and outlive others. For one thing, they are less likely to smoke, drink immoderately, abuse drugs, or engage in risky behaviors. They are more likely to take their vitamins, wear their seat belts, and follow their doctors' orders. Friedman also suggests that conscientious people are likely to enter into situations and relationships that are healthier. In regard to relationships, the finding is that being loved isn't as important as just having lots of people in one's life as well as caring for and helping others. It turns out that it really is better to give than to receive.

This research implies that it is critical to take care of the front third of your brain, which houses the prefrontal cortex and helps manage all of your decisions. Having a bigger, stronger prefrontal cortex helps you live longer because it is involved in conscientiousness, forethought, judgment, planning, organization, impulse control, empathy, and learning from mistakes. By the way, this is one of the major reasons for not letting children hit soccer balls with their heads and for thinking twice before allowing boys to play tackle football (hits to the head often cause injury to the brain—even if they don't cause a concussion).

Some of the other major findings reported from the study include the following:

- Hard work and accomplishment (often a sign of good brain function) are strong predictors of longevity. If you have been called a workaholic, but love what you do and balance it with healthy habits, keep doing it.
- Those who were most disappointed with their achievements died the youngest.
- Being unreliable and unsuccessful in careers (often a sign of poor brain function) had a whopping increase in mortality.
- Responding to loss with drinking, depression, anxiety and catastrophizing (further promoting poor brain function) was associated with early death. On the other hand, those who thrived after loss, following a period of grief and adjustment (using brain healthy habits), got a "resiliency bonus" and lived about five years longer than average.
- An optimistic, carefree attitude encouraged people to underestimate risks and approach their health in a lackadaisical fashion (behaviors associated with poor prefrontal cortex function and subsequent poor planning), thus decreasing longevity. Individuals with these traits died more often from accidents and avoidable deaths. Some in the media have erroneously interpreted this study to mean that pessimists live longer than optimists! This is not true. It is the optimists who work hard but who are also careful with their health who live longer than the average person. It is the carefree optimists—those who never worry, rarely plan or think about future consequences—who do not live as long.
- Thoughtful planning and perseverance (usually associated with good brain function) was associated with longevity.
- Prudent, persistent achievers with stable families and social support (all signs of healthy brain function) lived longer.
- People with habits, routines, and social networks which encouraged exercise did the best.
- Appropriate worry, meaning you care and think about the future, is important to stay healthy.

People who are conscientious and finish what they start seem to have a reduced risk of developing Alzheimer's disease, according to a twelve-year study involving Catholic nuns and priests. The most self-disciplined individuals were found to be 89 percent less likely to develop Alzheimer's disease than their peers.[24]

Brain Warriors recognize the importance of being conscientious. They assess their brains and bodies in five areas, as discussed in this chapter:

1. Brain Warriors assess their strategy.
2. Brain Warriors regularly assess their brains.
3. Brain Warriors assess and optimize their important health numbers.
4. Brain Warriors assess and strategically fight the war for health on multiple fronts.
5. Brain Warriors assess appropriate prevention strategies.

1.
BRAIN WARRIORS ASSESS THEIR STRATEGY

Brain Warriors assess and develop a health strategy they can execute wherever they are. Over the years we've been able to boil it down into three very simple steps:

- Brain envy
- Avoid anything that hurts the brain
- Engage in regular brain healthy habits

BRAIN ENVY

Freud was wrong. Penis envy is not the cause of most of your problems. Getting truly healthy starts with brain envy, which is when you care deeply about the health of your brain. Yet, most people rarely think about their brain because they can't see it. You can see the wrinkles in your skin or the fat around your belly and do something when you're unhappy with them, but the brain is different. Most people never look at it, and subsequently never think about caring for it.

BRAIN WARRIOR JEFF

Jeff is the CEO of a large, fast-growing marketing company. When he first came to see us Jeff was extremely fit on the outside. He was consistent in his workouts and wanted to keep his body healthy, but he had never really thought about his brain. Whenever he looked in the mirror he saw he was in great shape. Yet, his brain SPECT scan looked like it came from a much older man because of injuries Jeff had sustained years before and other habits that were not optimal. Seeing evidence of trouble on his scan, he immediately became a Brain Warrior and was much more serious about his brain's health. He significantly cut down his alcohol use, increased targeted supplements for his brain, and began mental workouts. Four months later his follow-up SPECT scan looked healthier and he had experienced better energy and cognitive clarity. He told an audience at a large national meeting that the first scan completely changed his perception about his brain and he started to really care about it, but the second scan, when he saw the improvement, motivated him even further to continue to pursue brain excellence.

AVOID ANYTHING THAT HURTS YOUR BRAIN

Any reputable martial arts sensei starts off new students by teaching them that the best way to win a fight is to avoid it in the first place. If you know a situation makes you vulnerable, stay away from it. Alcoholics who go to bars are asking for trouble. Drug addicts who drive by their dealer's home are likely to give in to temptation. Spending time with friends who eat poorly makes it much more likely you will do the same.

We often tell our Brain Warriors in Training to make one decision, not thirty. If you make the one decision to not buy ice cream at the grocery store, you do not have to make thirty decisions at home to not eat it as you pass by the freezer. If you make one decision to tell the waiter to take the bread off the table in a restaurant, you do not have to make thirty decisions over the course of a meal to not eat it.

Assess your vulnerable areas and look for ways to protect yourself from them. For example, if you give into temptation when you pass a certain fast-food restaurant—perhaps it has an emotional hook in your brain because your mother always took you there whenever you got good grades—consciously take a different route home so you're not tempted.

The table below lists many things that can damage your brain and body. We will expand on these items throughout the rest of this chapter and the book.

AVOID ANYTHING THAT HURTS YOUR BRAIN

Poor decisions
Brain injuries, concussions, and activities that put you at risk for them
Low physical activity
Cocaine, methamphetamines, inhalants, and other drugs of abuse
Marijuana
Too much alcohol
Many legal drugs, such as benzodiazepines, sleeping medications, and chronic pain medications
Smoking or chewing nicotine
Excessive caffeine (more than 100 milligrams a day)
Low blood sugar levels (associated with low prefrontal cortex function and impaired decision making)
High blood sugar levels (damages all organs)
Diabetes
Hypertension
Heart disease
Kidney or liver disease
Coronary artery bypass surgery
Cancer chemotherapy
General anesthesia (for some)
Chronic inflammation
Chronic stress
Insomnia
Sleep apnea
Standard American diet
Sugar
Fruit juice (high in sugar)
High omega-6 fatty acids
Low omega-3 fatty acids
Artificial food additives, dyes, and preservatives

Pesticides
Air pollution
Water pollution
Environmental toxins, such as mold and carbon monoxide
Infections, such as Lyme and HIV
Obesity
Gut inflammation
Exposure to heavy metals or poisonous chemicals
Oxygen deprivation
Untreated anxiety, depression, ADD, or PTSD
Vitamin and hormone deficiencies
High and low cholesterol
Gadget addiction
Negative thinking
Unhealthy peer group
Not knowing about the health of your brain

ENGAGE IN REGULAR BRAIN HEALTHY HABITS

Knowing what to do and what not to do is critical to success. The table below lists many things that are good for your brain and body. We will expand on these items throughout the rest of the book.

ENGAGE IN REGULAR BRAIN HEALTHY HABITS
Appropriate worry
Good decisions
Protecting your brain
Regular exercise
Healthy sports that require coordination and complex moves
    (dancing, table tennis, tennis, martial arts without head
    contact, golf, tai chi, qigong, yoga)
New learning
Daily motivation
Staying hydrated
Clean air
Stress management techniques
Basic supplements
Targeted supplements
Social support

Healthy weight
Sleeping 7 to 8 hours
Brain Warrior's Way nutrition program
    Anti-inflammatory
    Low-glycemic, high-fiber carbs
    Consistent protein
    Healthful fat
    Colorful foods
    Healing spices
Cautiously optimistic thinking
Meditation
Neurofeedback
Light therapy
Know the health of your brain
Have loving relationships
Healthy peer group
Passion and purpose

CHLOE'S GAME

We have been planting brain health in our children and grandchildren their whole lives. Since our youngest daughter, Chloe, was two years old, we have played a game with her we call "Chloe's Game." Subsequently, it has been played by children around the world, although it may be called "Amanda's Game" or "Justin's Game" in other households. It's based on one very simple question, "Is this good for my brain or bad for it?"

For example, if we said avocados, Chloe would gesture and say, "Two thumbs up, God's butter!"

If we say chocolate chip cookies, she'd usually say, "Thumbs down, too much sugar" (unless they were her mother's brain healthy cookie recipe).

If we said football, she'd say, "Two thumbs down; the brain is too soft to put it in a helmet and slam it up against other people."

If we said blueberries, she'd put her hands on her hips and ask, "Are they organic? Blueberries hold more pesticides than any other fruit. But organic blueberries are great. God's candy."

If her father says, "Talking back to your redheaded mother," she'll shake her head no and say, "Two thumbs down, way too much stress."

To be a Brain Warrior, you must love your brain, understand what to avoid because it hurts your brain, and know what to do to keep your brain healthy.

2.
BRAIN WARRIORS REGULARLY
ASSESS THEIR BRAINS

All of us need regular baseline brain health assessments. Unfortunately, this is rarely done for the brain. When Daniel turned fifty his doctor wanted him to have a colonoscopy. Daniel asked him why he didn't want to look at his brain. "Wasn't the other end of my body just as important?" From colonoscopies to mammograms, cardiac stress tests, Pap smears, and more, preventive screening and baseline testing are obtained for most organs, except for the most important organ—the one that runs your life.

At Amen Clinics we use brain SPECT imaging and quantitative electroencephalography (QEEG) to screen, evaluate, and help us diagnose our patients. These tools have revolutionized how we think about and treat our patients and inform virtually every aspect of how we help people. They give us biological data on the organ that makes decisions and runs your life.

A picture is worth a thousand words, but a map is worth a thousand pictures. A map tells you where you are and gives you directions on how to get to where you want to go. Without an accurate map you are lost, and it may cost you precious time in getting the help you need. We think of SPECT and QEEG as maps to help guide people to better brains and better lives.

Some of the important lessons learned from our brain imaging work are the following:

- Mild traumatic brain injuries are a major cause of psychiatric illness and many mental health professionals miss it in patients because they rarely look at the brains of their patients. Brain injuries are a major cause of drug and alcohol abuse, depression, anxiety, ADHD symptoms, suicide, and homelessness.
- Alzheimer's disease and other forms of dementia can be seen on SPECT scans years before people have symptoms. SPECT is a

leading indicator of problems, meaning it shows evidence of the disease process years before people show signs of it. Anatomical studies, such as CT and MRI, are lagging indicators. They show the problems later in the course of the illness, when interventions tend to be less effective.

- Functional brain imaging studies, such as with SPECT or QEEG, immediately decrease stigma for patients, because they help them see their problems as medical and not moral. This decreases the shame and guilt often associated with mental health issues. The images also help families become more supportive, and there is a heightened sense of compassion and forgiveness.

- Imaging completely changes the discussion around mental health. Quite frankly, few people really want to see a psychiatrist. Tana almost canceled her first date with Daniel when she found out he was a psychiatrist. No one wants to be labeled as defective or abnormal, but everyone wants a better brain. What if mental health was really brain health? The scans have taught us that lesson again and again.

- You are not stuck with the brain you have; you can make it better by using the program outlined in this book, and we have proven it on thousands of patients. This lesson drives our passion for this work. We have demonstrated we can help rehabilitate soldiers, professional football players, hockey players, police officers, and firefighters who have had brain damage as well as a host of other conditions.

KNOW YOUR BRAIN TYPE

Another important lesson we've learned at Amen Clinics is that all brains, even healthy ones, are not the same. When we first started to do our brain imaging work in 1991 we were looking for the one pattern that was associated with anxiety, depression, addictions, bipolar disorder, obsessive-compulsive disorder, autism, or ADD/ADHD. But we soon discovered there was not one brain pattern associated with any of these illnesses; they all had multiple types that require their own unique treatments. That made sense, because there will never be just one pattern for depression, because not all depressed people are the same. Some are withdrawn, others are angry, and still others are anxious or obsessive. Taking a one-size-fits-all approach invites failure and frustration. Symptom-guided treatment is often ineffective and harmful.

The scans helped us understand the type of anxiety, depression, ADD, obesity, or addiction a person had, so we could better target treatment to individual brains. This one idea led to a dramatic breakthrough in our own personal effectiveness with patients, and it opened up a new world of understanding and hope for the tens of thousands of people who have come to see us and the millions of people who have read our books or seen our shows. In previously published books, Daniel has written about seven types of ADD, seven types of anxiety and depression, six types of addictions, and five types of overeaters. Understanding these types is critical to getting the right help, because each of the disorder subtypes requires a different treatment plan.

Here is a summary of some of the common brain types.

Brain Type 1: Balanced

People with this type tend to have healthy brains overall, which allows them to

- Be focused
- Be flexible
- Be positive
- Be relaxed

Overall, their moods are stable and they are consistent and positive. Traits that come from a healthy brain.

Brain Type 2: Spontaneous

People with this type tend to

- Be spontaneous
- Take risks
- Be creative, with out-of-the-box thinking
- Be restless
- Be easily distracted
- Be focused only when very interested

The SPECT scans of Spontaneous brain type people typically have lower activity in the front part of the brain called the prefrontal cortex (PFC). Think of the PFC as the brain's brake. It stops us from saying or doing things that are not in our best interest, but it can also stop creative thinking. The PFC is the little voice in our heads that helps us decide between the banana and the banana split. The Spontaneous brain type tends to be associated with lower dopamine levels in the brain, which may cause people to be more restless, take more risks, and need to be very interested in something in order to stay focused.

Our research team has published several studies showing that when Spontaneous brain type people try to concentrate, they actually have less activity in the PFC, which causes them to need excitement or stimulation in order to focus (think of firefighters and race car drivers). Smokers and heavy coffee drinkers also tend to fit this type, as they use these substances to turn their brains on.

The Spontaneous brain type is best optimized by boosting dopamine levels to strengthen the PFC. Higher-protein, lower-carbohydrate diets tend to help, as do physical exercise and certain stimulating supplements, such as green tea, rhodiola, and ginseng. Any supplement or medicine that calms the brain, such as 5-hydroxytryptophan (5-HTP) and selective serotonin reuptake inhibitors (SSRIs), may make this type worse. These substances lower the already low PFC function, which can then take the brakes off behavior. For example, we have treated many people who had done things they later regretted, such as becoming hypersexual or spending money they did not have while they were taking SSRIs. It turned out they had low activity in the PFC, and the serotonin-boosting medications diminished their judgment.

Brain Type 3: Persistent

People with this type tend to

- Be persistent
- Be relentless or strong willed
- Like things a certain way
- Get stuck on thoughts
- Hold on to hurts
- See what is wrong in themselves or others

People with a Persistent brain type are often take-charge people who won't take no for an answer. They tend to be tenacious and stubborn. In addition, they may worry, have trouble sleeping, be argumentative and oppositional, and hold grudges. The Persistent brain type often has increased activity in the front part of the brain called the anterior cingulate gyrus (ACG). We think of the ACG as the brain's gear shifter. It helps people go from thought to thought or move from action to action. It is involved with being mentally flexible and going with the flow. When the ACG is overactive, usually due to low levels of serotonin, people can have problems shifting attention, which can make them persist, even when it may not be a good idea for them to do so. Caffeine and diet pills tend to make this type worse, because this brain type does *not* need more stimulation, and people who have this type may need a glass of wine at night, or two or three, to calm their worries.

The best strategy to balance the Persistent brain type is to find natural ways to boost serotonin because it is calming to the brain. Physical exercise boosts serotonin as does using certain supplements, such as 5-HTP and saffron. High-glycemic carbohydrates turn to sugar quickly and increase serotonin, which is why many people become addicted to simple carbohydrates like bread, pasta, and sweets. These are "mood foods" and are often used to self-medicate an underlying mood issue. Avoid these quick fixes because they can cause long-term health problems.

Brain Type 4: Sensitive

People with this type tend to

- Be sensitive
- Feel deeply
- Be empathic
- Struggle with moods
- Be pessimistic
- Struggle with negative thoughts

SPECT scans of the Sensitive brain type tend to show increased activity in the limbic or emotional centers of the brain, making these individuals sensitive, empathic, and deeply feeling but also subject to issues with their moods. They may also struggle with being more pessimistic and having negative thoughts.

Exercise, omega-3 fatty acids, and certain supplements, such as SAMe and vitamin D, can help the Sensitive brain type. If someone with this type is also a Persistent brain type, supplements or medications that boost serotonin may help best with mood and worry.

Brain Type 5: Cautious

People with this type tend to

- Be prepared
- Be cautious
- Be motivated
- Be reserved
- Be busy-minded
- Be restless

On SPECT images of individuals with a Cautious brain type, we often see heightened activity in the anxiety centers of the brain, such as the basal ganglia, insular cortex, or amygdala. Often, due to low levels of the neurotransmitter gamma-aminobutyric acid (GABA), people with this type of brain tend to struggle more with anxiety, which causes them to be more cautious and reserved, but on the flip side, they are also more prepared.

Soothing this type with meditation and hypnosis can help them feel more balanced, as can a combination of vitamin B_6, magnesium, and GABA.

It is common to have more than one brain type and when we look at all of the potential combinations it adds up to sixteen types, such as Spontaneous-Persistent-Sensitive or Sensitive-Cautious. Many years ago we realized that not everyone can come to one of our clinics to get scanned, so based on thousands of scans, Daniel developed a questionnaire that helps predict what the scans might look like. The questionnaire is not as good as actually looking at the brain, but it is still helpful and used by thousands of medical and mental health professionals around the world. You can find out your brain type as part of our free Brain Health Assessment on amenclinics.com, where you'll also find specific suggestions to help each type.

BRAIN FIT WEBNEURO

In addition to our questionnaire and brain imaging work, we also test the brain function of our patients and clients using a sophisticated online computerized neuropsychological test called Brain Fit WebNeuro, which measures a wide range of cognitive and emotional functions. It takes about 35 minutes to complete and provides an objective assessment of how your brain works in fourteen specific areas, scoring each one on a scale of 1 to 10. The test also generates an overall brain health score.

BRAIN FIT WEBNEURO MEASURES

1. Motor coordination
2. Processing speed
3. Attention
4. Flexibility
5. Inhibition (self-control)
6. Memory
7. Executive function (judgment)
8. Stress
9. Anxiety
10. Mood
11. Ability to read faces
12. Emotional resilience
13. Social capacity
14. Positivity or negativity bias

The test gives clear baseline information that allows us to recommend targeted exercises and fun brain games to strengthen your vulnerable areas. Knowing the health of your brain with baseline testing is a critical strategy to keeping it strong over the long run. We want you to repeat Brain Fit WebNeuro every few months to see if you are making your desired progress. You can sign up to take the test at mybrainfitlife.com.

New research shows that lower memory and thinking scores on cognitive tests obtained up to eighteen years earlier can indicate possible Alzheimer's disease later on.[25] How concerned are you about your brain health? How good would it feel to know you don't have a problem? Or, if you do have a problem, to know there are things you can do about it? All of us need baseline testing and regular checkups to pick up any problems early, when treatment is most likely to be effective.

3.
BRAIN WARRIORS ASSESS AND OPTIMIZE
THEIR IMPORTANT HEALTH NUMBERS

The important business management principle, "You cannot change what you do not measure," also applies to your health numbers. Following is a list of important health numbers you should know. Work to optimize, not just normalize, them on an ongoing basis. Who wants to be normal? Fifty percent of people age eighty-five and older will be diagnosed with Alzheimer's disease. That's normal and we want no part of it and neither should you.

BODY MASS INDEX (BMI)

Body mass index, or BMI, is a measure of weight compared to height. An optimal BMI is between 18.5 and 25, the overweight range falls between 25 and 30, over 30 indicates obesity, and over 40 indicates morbid obesity. When you take our free Brain Health Assessment on amenclinics.com it calculates your BMI. Knowing this number is important because being overweight or obese is associated with less brain volume and lower brain activity. Plus obesity increases the risk for Alzheimer's disease[26] and depression.[27] With two-thirds of Americans overweight, this is the biggest brain drain in the history of our country. It is critical to get your weight under control, and knowing your BMI prevents you from lying to yourself.[28] In our experience, when you get your weight under control, you can reverse the damage to your brain. Follow the strategies in this book to get your BMI to optimal levels.

BRAIN WARRIORS MARK AND DEBBIE

Mark and Debbie are close friends. One day Mark, a pastoral psychologist and world leader in the field of addiction medicine, and Daniel were speaking at a conference together. When they were at dinner Mark seemed totally oblivious to what he ordered, even though he was overweight and had diabetes. This concerned Daniel, and even more so when he saw Mark inject himself with insulin at the table.

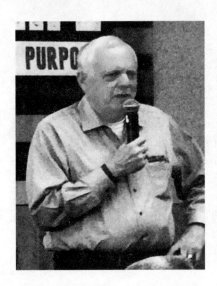 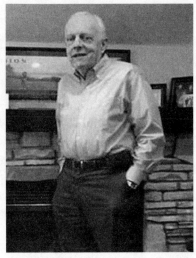

Without making a big fuss, Daniel asked Mark how tall he was.

"Six feet," Mark said.

"How much do you weigh?" was Daniel's next question.

"Two hundred forty-four pounds," he answered.

Using the calculator on his phone, Daniel determined Mark's BMI. His score was 33. "You are in the obese range, my friend, and not by a little bit. I am worried about you," Daniel said softly.

"You are so cold," Mark replied, with a bit of anxiety in his voice.

"Not as cold as you are going to be six feet under if you don't get your health and weight under control," Daniel said, now with a dead-serious tone in his voice. "Know the truth and the truth will set you free."

The word *obese* really got Mark's attention. The next month he lost 10 pounds. Two years later he was down 53 pounds and had increased focus, energy, memory, and sexual ability. What's more, he had cut his insulin dosage in half. His wife, Debbie, is a zealot for her health and Mark's. They became Brain Warriors together, and the mutual support allows them, in their mid-sixties, to have a much better quality of life than they did even thirty years earlier.

Mark and Debbie told us some of the things they did together to encourage their joint success:

- Celebrating the attainment of their mutual weight loss goals
- Studying menus and asking clear, polite questions to waiters about ingredients

- Making a list of their favorite restaurants where they knew the food is "safe"
- Shopping for blenders and food processors to make their own shakes
- Shopping the perimeter of grocery stores for fresh, healthful food
- Cooking together for the first time in their marriage
- Studying cookbooks, mainly Tana's, for inspiration
- Noticing the effects of food and sleep on their mood and energy
- Shopping together for new clothes

We asked Mark if being a Brain Warrior was hard. He laughed, saying, "Being sick is hard. Having brain fog, fatigue, and a low libido is hard. This is easy. I'll never go back. Thank you for caring enough about me to have that hard conversation."

WAIST TO HEIGHT RATIO (WHtR)

Another way to measure the health of your weight is with your waist to height ratio (WHtR). WHtR is calculated by dividing waist size by height. For example, a person with a 32-inch waist who is 70 inches tall (5 foot 10) would divide 32 by 70 to get a WHtR of 45.7 percent. Generally speaking, it's healthy for your waist size to be half your height or less in inches. When measuring your waist size, you actually have to use a tape measure! Don't hazard a guess or rely on your pants size, which can vary between manufacturers. In our experience, 90 percent of people will underestimate their waist circumference. Get an accurate measurement.

Some researchers believe this number is even more accurate than BMI because the most dangerous place to carry weight is in the abdomen. Abdominal fat, which is associated with a larger waist, is metabolically active and produces various hormones that can cause harmful health effects, such as diabetes, elevated blood pressure, and high cholesterol and triglyceride levels.

BLOOD PRESSURE

Good blood pressure is critical for brain health. High blood pressure and even blood pressure at the higher end of the normal range (prehypertension) is associated with lower overall brain function,[29] which means more bad decisions. According to the CDC about 70 million Americans—one-third of the population—have hypertension and another one-third has prehypertension.[30] Being hypertensive is the second leading preventable cause of death and is associated with heart disease and stroke. Here are the numbers you should know.

OPTIMAL

- Systolic 90–120
- Diastolic 60–80

PREHYPERTENSIVE

- Systolic 120–139
- Diastolic 80–89

HYPERTENSIVE

- Systolic 140 and higher
- Diastolic 90 and higher

HYPOTENSIVE—TOO LOW CAN ALSO BE A PROBLEM

- Systolic 90 or lower
- Diastolic 60 or lower

Check your blood pressure or have your doctor check it on a regular basis. If your blood pressure is abnormal, take it seriously. Strategies that can help lower your blood pressure include

- Losing weight
- Daily exercise
- Reducing sugar and sodium intake
- Eating foods high in omega-3 fatty acids
- Deep-breathing exercises and meditation to lower stress
- Eating potassium-rich foods, such as dark leafy greens, broccoli, pork, tilapia, baked acorn squash, sweet potatoes, quinoa, avocados, wild mushrooms, red bell peppers, bananas, kiwi, white beans
- Eliminating caffeine
- Focusing on getting at least 7 hours of sleep at night
- Optimizing your vitamin D level
- Medication, if needed

GET KEY LABORATORY TESTS

Laboratory tests will provide another set of important numbers to know. Ask your health-care professional to order them or you can order them for yourself at websites like saveonlabs.com. If your numbers are abnormal, please work with your healthcare professional to get them into optimal ranges. Here are the key lab tests you should know.

Complete Blood Count (CBC)

The CBC is a test that checks the health of your blood, including red and white blood cells. People with a low red blood cell count can feel anxious, tired, and have significant memory problems. Large red blood cells may mean you are drinking too much alcohol. A high level of white blood cells may indicate infection. Check with your health-care provider for treatment suggestions.

General Metabolic Panel with Fasting Blood Sugar and Lipid Panel

A fasting blood test, which checks your metabolism, blood sugar, and lipid levels, checks the health of your liver and kidneys, risk of diabetes, cholesterol, and triglycerides.

Knowing your fasting blood sugar level is especially important.

- Normal is between 70 and 100 milligrams per deciliter (mg/dL).
- Optimal is between 70 and 89 mg/dL.
- Prediabetes is between 100 and 125 mg/dL.
- Diabetes is 126 mg/dL or higher.

Why is high fasting blood sugar a problem? High blood sugar causes vascular (blood vessel) problems throughout your whole body, including your brain. Over time, it causes blood vessels to become brittle and vulnerable to breakage. High blood sugar leads not only to diabetes but also to heart disease, strokes, visual impairment, impaired wound healing, wrinkled skin, and cognitive problems. Diabetes doubles the risk for Alzheimer's disease. According to a large study from Kaiser Permanente, for every point above 85 mg/dL, patients had an additional 6 percent increased risk of developing diabetes in the following ten years.

For example, 86 mg/dL means a 6 percent increased risk, 87 mg/dL means a 12 percent increased risk, and so on. Those who had a fasting blood sugar above 90 mg/dL already had vascular damage and were at risk for having damage to the kidneys and eyes. Strategies to lower fasting blood sugar are discussed in the next section, "Hemoglobin A_{1c} (HbA_{1c})."

Cholesterol and triglycerides are also important, especially because 60 percent of the solid weight of the brain is fat. Cholesterol that is either too high or too low is bad for the brain. According to the American Heart Association, normal levels are as follows:

- Total cholesterol should be between 135 and 200 mg/dL. (Note that levels below 160 mg/dL have been associated with depression, suicide, homicide, and death from all causes, so we think optimal is between 160 and 200 mg/dL.)
- High-density lipoprotein (HDL) should be 60 mg/dL or higher.
- Low-density lipoprotein (LDL) should be 100 mg/dL or lower.
- Triglycerides should be below 100 mg/dL.

Knowing the particle size of your LDL cholesterol (your health-care professional can order this test) is important because large particles are less toxic than small particles. If cholesterol is a concern for you, we recommend *The Great Cholesterol Myth* by Jonny Bowden and Stephen Sinatra.

To optimize your cholesterol levels consider the following strategies:

- Eliminate added sugars and refined carbohydrates from your diet.
- Eat foods high in soluble fiber.
- Increase your vegetable intake.
- Eat foods high in omega-3 fatty acids.
- Exercise regularly.
- Stop smoking.
- Lose weight if you're overweight.
- Check with your physician about taking niacin, plant sterols, or other cholesterol-lowering supplements or medications.

Hemoglobin A$_{1c}$ (HbA$_{1c}$)

The HbA$_{1c}$ test shows your average blood sugar levels over the previous two to three months and is used to diagnose diabetes and prediabetes. Normal results for a nondiabetic person are in the range of 4 to 5.6 percent, optimal is under 5.3 percent. Prediabetes is indicated by levels in the 5.7 to 6.4 percent range. Higher numbers may indicate diabetes. Strategies to lower your HbA$_{1c}$ include the following:

- The nutrition advice given in Part 3, especially eliminating sugar and refined carbohydrates and adding protein and healthy fat at every meal.
- Losing weight if you're overweight.
- Exercising regularly.
- Taking supplements, such as chromium, alpha-lipoic acid, and cinnamon.
- Checking with your physician to see if other treatment is necessary.

Vitamin D

Low levels of vitamin D have been associated with obesity,[31] depression,[32] cognitive impairment,[33] heart disease,[34] reduced immunity,[35] cancer,[36] psychosis,[37] and all causes of mortality.[38] The blood test to get is 25-hydroxyvitamin D level. A normal vitamin D level is between 30 and 100 nanograms per deciliter (ng/dL), with the most optimal range between 50 and 80 ng/dL. If your vitamin D level is low, get more sunshine in a safe way and/or take a vitamin D$_3$ supplement and check your level again in three months. Two-thirds of the U.S. population is low in vitamin D—the same percentage of citizens who are overweight or obese. According to one study, when vitamin D levels are low, the hormone leptin that tells you to stop eating is not effective. One of the reasons for the dramatic rise in vitamin D deficiency is that people are wearing more sunscreen when outside and spending more time inside while working or sitting in front of the television or computer.

Thyroid Panel

Abnormal thyroid hormone levels are a common cause of anxiety, depression, forgetfulness, weight problems, and lethargy. Having low thyroid levels decreases overall brain activity, which can impair your thinking, judgment, and self-control. Low thyroid functioning can make it nearly impossible to manage weight effectively. High levels are associated with anxiety, insomnia, and feeling agitated. The following thyroid indicators should be checked:

- Thyroid stimulating hormone (TSH); normal levels are between 0.4 and 3.0 International Units per liter (IU/L).
- Free T_3; check with your lab for normal ranges.
- Free T_4; check with your lab for normal ranges.
- Thyroid antibodies (thyroid peroxidase and thyroglobulin antibodies); check with your lab for normal ranges.

Unfortunately, there is no single symptom or test result that will properly diagnose low thyroid function (hypothyroidism). The key is to gather your symptoms and your blood test results and consult with your physician. Symptoms of low thyroid include fatigue, depression, mental fog, dry skin, hair loss (especially the outer third of your eyebrows), feeling cold when others feel normal, constipation, hoarse voice, and weight gain.

C-Reactive Protein (CRP)

Your level of C-reactive protein is a measure of inflammation. Inflammation, which comes from the Latin word for "fire," is associated with many chronic illnesses, including depression, dementia, and pain syndromes.[39] When CRP is high, it is as if you had a low-level fire in your body destroying your organs. A healthy range is between 0.0 and 1.0 mg/dL.

Fat cells produce chemicals that increase inflammation, which is a pressing reason to monitor weight and belly fat. The most common cause of elevated C-reactive protein is metabolic syndrome or insulin resistance. The second most common cause is sensitivity to food, such as gluten. High CRP levels can also indicate hidden infections. Other strategies to lower CRP levels include the following:

- Quit smoking.
- Eat an anti-inflammatory Brain Warrior diet.
- Exercise regularly.
- Be sure to get 7 to 8 hours of sleep a night.
- Whittle your waistline (the goal for women is less than 35 inches; for men, less than 40 inches)
- Reduce stress.
- Eat foods rich in omega-3 fatty acids.

Homocysteine

Elevated homocysteine levels (more than 10 micromoles/liter), checked via a blood test, are associated with atherosclerosis (hardening and narrowing of the arteries) and an increased risk of heart attacks, strokes, blood clot formation, and possibly Alzheimer's disease. Homocysteine is a sensitive marker for a folate deficiency. Strategies to lower homocysteine include the following:

- Adding more folate-rich foods to your diet, such as fruits, green leafy vegetables, beans, and lentils.
- Losing weight if you're overweight.
- Avoiding too much alcohol.
- Eliminating smoking.
- Reducing stress.
- Eating foods high in omega-3 fatty acids.
- Being sure to get enough vitamin B_6 (25 milligrams), B_{12} (500 micrograms), and folate (400 to 800 micrograms).

Ferritin

Checking the blood for ferritin measures your body's iron stores. High levels are associated with inflammation and insulin resistance. Low levels are associated with anemia, restless legs, ADD, and low motivation and low energy. Levels between 15 to 100 ng/mL are ideal. Women often have lower iron stores than men, due to blood loss from menstruation. Some theorize that this is one of the reasons women tend to live longer than men. If your level is low, consider taking iron. If it is high, donating blood may help.

Free and Total Serum Testosterone

For both men and women, low levels of testosterone have been associated with low energy, cardiovascular disease, obesity, low libido, depression, and Alzheimer's disease. The levels are checked via a blood test. Normal levels for adult males are as follows:

- Total testosterone should be between 280 and 800 ng/dL; optimal is 500 to 800 ng/dL.
- Free testosterone should be between 7.2 and 24 picograms per milliliter (pg/mL; optimal 12 to 24 pg/mL).

Normal levels for adult females are as follows:

- Total testosterone should be between 6 and 82 ng/dL; optimal is 40 to 82 ng/dL.
- Free testosterone should be between 0.0 and 2.2 pg/mL; optimal is 1.0 to 2.2 pg/mL.

To naturally optimize your testosterone levels:

- Eliminate all sugar and refined carbohydrates.
- Exercise, including weight lifting.
- Consider checking your dehydroepiandrosterone (DHEA) level and taking a DHEA supplement if your level is low.
- Check with your physician about hormone replacement.

Estrogen and Progesterone for Women

Depending on the circumstances, estrogen and progesterone are measured in blood or saliva. Menstruating women are usually tested on day twenty-one of their cycles, and postmenopausal women can be measured anytime. Estrogen is responsible for vaginal lubrication, helps with libido and memory—and so much more. Progesterone calms emotions, contributes to restful sleep, and acts as a diuretic.

Knowing and optimizing these numbers is critical to helping your brain work right. If any of them are abnormal, the function of your brain can be troubled too. Work with your local health-care provider to help get these numbers into the most optimal range possible.

4.
BRAIN WARRIORS ASSESS AND STRATEGICALLY FIGHT THE WAR FOR HEALTH ON MULTIPLE FRONTS

Your brain gets sick or it ages in many different ways, and that is exactly how we assess and optimize it. Assessing and targeting multiple processes like inflammation, blood flow, gut health, blood sugar levels, and more can make a radical difference in your health. Single-mechanism interventions, such as taking just single supplements like ginkgo or vitamin E by themselves, have not consistently worked in large-scale studies to stave off cognitive impairment. But when we use smart combinations to fight the war for brain health on multiple fronts our effectiveness significantly improves.

For example, we typically use the following nutrients in a multiple-mechanism approach:

- Omega-3 fatty acids to decrease overall inflammation
- Ginkgo to support healthy cerebral blood flow
- Probiotics to support gut health
- Alpha-lipoic acid to help stabilize blood sugar levels and protect against nerve cell damage
- Vitamins B, C, and D for nutrient loading
- Huperzine A and choline to boost acetylcholine levels, one of the main amino acids involved with learning and memory
- Phosphatidylserine for nerve cell membrane fluidity
- N-acetyl-cysteine (NAC) for antioxidant support and detoxification

This is exactly what we did at Amen Clinics when we performed the first and largest brain imaging and rehabilitation study on active and retired NFL players. We saw significant improvement in 80 percent of players.

BRAIN WARRIORS TACKLE FOOTBALL, FIND HOPE

Brain Warrior Anthony Davis

In July 2007, Anthony Davis came to see us as a patient. AD, as his friends call him, is a College Football Hall of Fame running back from the University of Southern California who played professional football for eight years. He was concerned about his own memory issues and the cognitive problems he saw in other retired NFL players. His brain showed clear evidence of trauma to his prefrontal cortex and left temporal lobe. Within five months of being on a program of supplements targeting multiple mechanisms, such as inflammation, blood flow, blood sugar stabilization, antioxidant support, and nutrient loading, AD reported improvements in memory, energy, focus, and judgment—and his brain was better.

As AD improved, he started to tell other active and retired players that brain rehabilitation may be possible. In January 2009, AD asked Daniel to speak to the Los Angeles chapter of the NFL's Retired Players Association. Daniel was horrified by the level of depression and dementia present at the meeting. One player asked him the same question six times. At a time when the NFL seemed to be in denial about the issue, an independent group needed to answer the question about brain damage and football. Our research team at Amen Clinics decided to tackle the issue with the help of the Los Angeles chapter. Over the next year we recruited more than a hundred active and former NFL players. The results were clear: Playing professional football was associated with long-term brain damage.

Once we identified the damage, we wanted to see if we could improve damaged brains. The exciting answer was yes. In a published study, we demonstrated that 80 percent of our players showed clinically significant improvement, especially increased blood flow to the prefrontal cortex and temporal lobes, as well as improvements in memory, mood, sleep, and motivation, using the same program we used with AD.[40] One of our players, former Los Angeles Ram and actor Fred Dryer, wrote, "With the program I have replaced a part of me that over time had slowly slipped away."

Let's dive deeper into three of these mechanisms: blood flow, inflammation, and gut health.

BLOOD FLOW

Blood flow is essential to life. Blood brings nutrients to your cells and takes away toxins. New research suggests that brain cells do not age as fast as we thought. The blood vessels that feed neurons are what ages.[41] If you want to keep your brain healthy, it is critical to protect your blood vessels. Because the brain uses 20 percent of the blood flow in your body, we like to say, "Whatever is good for your heart is good for your brain, and whatever is bad for your heart is also bad for your brain." In 2007, when Daniel wrote *The Brain in Love*, he realized he was missing a very important piece of the puzzle, and subsequently says, "Whatever is good for your heart is good for your brain is good for your genitals. And whatever is bad for your heart is bad for your brain is bad for your genitals. It is all about blood flow." As erectile dysfunction is skyrocketing (just turn on the television and you'll be bombarded with commercials for Viagra, Levitra, and Cialis), so are brain problems. According to the Massachusetts Male Aging Study 40 percent of forty-year-old men have erectile dysfunction, which means 40 percent of forty-year-old men also have brain dysfunction. With age, the rate increases to a frightening level. The same study reported that 70 percent of seventy-year-old men had erectile dysfunction, which means that 70 percent of seventy-year-old men likely also have brain dysfunction.[42]

In this context, blood flow envy (a new way to think of penis envy) seems appropriate. To keep your brain healthy it is critical to focus on strengthening vascular health. To do this it takes three strategies:

1. Develop blood flow envy; you have to care about your blood vessels.
2. Avoid things that hurt vascular health, such as stress, caffeine, and nicotine (the latter two constrict blood flow to the brain and other organs). Get treatment for coronary artery disease, heart arrhythmias, prediabetes and diabetes, prehypertension and hypertension, poor sleep, sleep apnea, and drug and alcohol abuse.

3. Do things to help strengthen your blood vessels, such as stress management, Brain Warrior nutrition, hydration, great sleep habits, and supplements such as gingko biloba, and omega-3 fatty acids.

INFLAMMATION

Just as poor blood flow is devastating to brain function so is chronic inflammation. Inflammation is your body's way of coping with injury or "insult." It is a vital biological response that your body must be able to elicit in the right balance at the right time. You would never want to completely eliminate your ability to create inflammation because you wouldn't heal properly. When you're injured or you develop an infection, the many functions of your immune system—both innate (what you're born with) and adaptive (what you've acquired)—jump into action and set off an acute inflammatory reaction. A cascade of events occurs: Blood vessels dilate, blood flow to the affected area increases, and pro-inflammatory immune cells and proteins rush to the scene. Nearby tissue becomes swollen, warm, and red as the immune system "inflames" the area and fights to destroy bacteria, eliminate toxins, and clear the way for the healing process to begin.

However, injury and infection aren't the only things that trigger inflammation. Environmental toxins, hormone imbalances, emotional stress, excess body fat—especially belly fat—and high blood sugar, along with certain kinds of pro-inflammatory foods, also cause inflammation. This type of inflammation, even though it's at a low level, is not helpful, because it is chronic—that is, it stays turned on indefinitely, rather than just occasionally when an injury or infection occurs.

Over time, chronic inflammation damages your body and contributes to a range of diseases, including heart disease, arthritis, gastrointestinal disorders, cancer, Alzheimer's disease, and high blood pressure.

The standard American diet is filled with many pro-inflammatory foods, including sugar; high-glycemic, low-fiber carbohydrates; transfats; and excessive omega-6 fatty acids. To decrease inflammation, pay attention to your Brain Warrior Nutrition, especially consuming omega-3 fatty acids from fish, nuts, cooked broccoli, and avocados. Green tea and cocoa can be helpful, as can certain spices such as curcumin, rosemary, and garlic. To decrease inflammation it is also critical to take care of your gums and avoid periodontal disease.

Flossing your teeth is a brain exercise!

HEAL YOUR GUT TO BOOST YOUR BRAIN

The gut is often called the second brain. It is loaded with nervous tissue and it is in direct communication with the brain between your ears, which is why we get butterflies when we get excited or have loose bowels when upset. Anxiety, depression, stress, and grief all express themselves with emotional pain, and quite often, gastrointestinal distress.

Your gut is one of the most important organs for the health of your brain. It is estimated that the gastrointestinal tract is loaded with about 100 trillion microorganisms (bacteria, yeast, and others), about ten times the total number of cells in the human body. To be healthy, the relationship of good bugs to bad bugs needs to be positively skewed—around 85 percent good to 15 percent troublemakers. When the balance is tipped the other way, all sorts of physical and mental problems can arise. Keeping your gut in proper balance is essential to your mental health.[43]

There is new evidence that friendly gut bacteria actually deter invading troublemakers, such as *E.coli*, and help us withstand stress. If the good bugs are deficient, either from a poor diet that feeds yeast overgrowth (such as from sugar) or the excessive presence of antibiotics (even as far back as childhood) that killed the good bacteria, we are more likely to feel anxious, stressed, and depressed.

The greatest danger from antibiotics does not come from those prescribed by your doctor, but rather from the foods you eat. The prevalence of antibiotics found in conventionally raised meats and dairy has the potential to throw off the balance of good to bad bacteria. It is estimated that 70 percent of the total antibiotic use in the United States is for livestock, which is why it is critical to eat antibiotic- and hormone-free meats whenever possible.

Disorders ranging from ADD to autism, depression, and schizophrenia have been connected to intestinal bacteria imbalances that increase gut permeability. The intestines provide an important barrier to the outside world. If the gut becomes too permeable, often called "leaky gut," inflammation and illness can be created throughout the body. Optimizing the health of your gut is critical to your mental health. Here are some factors that decrease healthy gut bacteria:

- Medications (antibiotics, oral contraceptives, proton pump inhibitors, steroids, nonsteroidal anti-inflammatory drugs)
- Sugar intake
- Artificial sweeteners
- Bactericidal chemicals in water
- Pesticide residues in food
- Alcohol
- Stress, including physiological, emotional, and environmental
- Radiation
- High-intensity exercise, such as marathons

What does this mean for you? Follow the brain healthy food guidelines in Part 3, especially by eliminating most of the simple sugars from your diet that feed the bad bugs. Focus on eating smart carbohydrates (low glycemic, high fiber), which enhance healthy gut flora. Also, consider taking a daily probiotic to give the good bugs a head start. Be careful with antibiotics, and if you have had a lot of them in the past, a probiotic and a healthy diet become even more important to the health of your brain.

5.
BRAIN WARRIORS ASSESS APPROPRIATE PREVENTION STRATEGIES

Any warrior knows that avoiding a fight or preventing trouble is just as important as winning a battle. Brain health is no different. New research shows you can decrease your risk of Alzheimer's disease and other forms of dementia by 60 percent or more and those same strategies will help your mood, focus, and memory.

Dementia is defined as damage to brain cells that results in progressive thinking and memory problems. Dementia is the umbrella category; Alzheimer's disease is only one of the types, along with alcoholic dementia, Parkinson's dementia, frontal temporal lobe dementia, and vascular dementia, among others.

DEMENTIA IS THE UMBRELLA CATEGORY

Alzheimer's disease
Vascular dementia
Frontal temporal lobe dementia
Lewy body dementia often associated with Parkinson's disease
Alcohol-related dementia
Infectious disease causes
Toxic causes
Chronic traumatic encephalopathy
Cognitive changes caused by depression

Leslie was fifty-four years old when she first came to see us. She was always worried about her mother, who had Alzheimer's disease, and constantly on guard to protect her mother from wandering off. Subsequently, Leslie became depressed and had developed sleeping and memory problems from the chronic stress. One of Leslie's first questions was, "What can I do to decrease my chances of getting Alzheimer's? I never want my kids going through this stress." We told Leslie the same thing we are going to tell you:

The best strategy to decrease your risk of accelerated aging, Alzheimer's disease, and other forms of dementia is to eliminate all of the risk factors that are associated with them—and the good news is that most of them are either preventable or treatable. A 2015 review of many studies reported that there were nine modifiable risk factors that explained two-thirds of Alzheimer's disease cases.[44]

1. Obesity
2. Low educational attainment
3. Depression
4. High blood pressure

5. Carotid artery narrowing
6. Frailty
7. Smoking
8. High homocysteine level
9. Type 2 diabetes

In the following sections we show you which risk factors you must attack to help stave off dementia and premature aging. If you have depression or dementia in your family, you need to start prevention as early as possible. You want to start now.

Obesity, Diabetes, Hypertension, and Heart Disease

Obesity, diabetes, hypertension, and heart disease all increase your risk for both depression and dementia. You have to take your physical health seriously because it directly affects your brain and, after just a short period of time, these illnesses decrease blood flow to your brain, which in turn decreases your focus, energy, memory, and the ability to make good decisions.[45] In a study from Russia, scientists looked at twenty-four patients with metabolic syndrome (MetS), including obesity, hypertension, and high blood sugar. This study demonstrated all patients with MetS showed lower blood flow in all regions of the brain compared with a healthy group. The patients' attention and memory scores were lower by 25 percent and 22 percent, respectively, compared with the control group. After six months of treatment to lower their blood pressure, patients showed increased blood flow and improved attention and visual memory.[46] Another study from Newcastle University showed that type 2 diabetes could be reversed by getting your weight under control.[47]

OBESOGENS (ENVIRONMENTAL FACTORS THAT INTERFERE WITH WEIGHT LOSS) TO AVOID

- Bisphenol A (BPA)
- Processed foods
- High-fructose corn syrup
- Pesticides
- Teflon

Low Estrogen, Testosterone, and Thyroid

Low estrogen, testosterone, and thyroid levels increase your risk of both dementia and depression. We seem to be biologically programmed to die after our children are raised in order to save on the earth's resources, which may be why our hormone levels drop significantly in our fifties. We don't know about you, but we are not okay with that. We are just getting started and love the wisdom of age, but we need our bodies and brains to be healthy to feel vibrant. Plus grandchildren are just way too much fun! You need to know your hormone levels and work to optimize them, as mentioned earlier.

Tobacco, Drug, and Alcohol Abuse

Smoking and drug and alcohol abuse increase your risk for dementia, so if these are a problem for you, stopping immediately decreases these risk factors. In our offices we usually have orchids because of how amazing they are. We often ask our patients, if the orchids become damaged by being exposed to toxins in the soil, how do we bring them back to health? First, we have to eliminate the toxins and give the orchids the highest-quality nutrients possible. Your brain is the same way. We are disturbed by the recent societal messages about marijuana and alcohol. These are not health foods. Marijuana use has doubled from 2001 to 2013.[48]

No doubt, some parts of the marijuana plant can be helpful to increase appetite and may help with pain, glaucoma and seizure control. When Tana's stepfather died of painful pancreatic cancer, we were glad he had access to medical marijuana. But as Daniel has published, marijuana is associated with lower overall blood flow and has a toxic effect on many brains.[49] We have also seen marijuana associated with coordination difficulties, learning issues, lack of motivation, and memory problems. When we posted the marijuana image below, it blew up our social media pages with passionate discussions on either side of the argument. All we can say is that our clinical experience with marijuana is twenty-six years long, and we have scanned thousands of users. Overall, it does not make the brain look healthier. Is it worse than alcohol or other legal drugs like Xanax? No. And it usually doesn't make people violent, like alcohol can. Should we incarcerate people who smoke pot? We think it is a really bad idea to put them with criminals, in chronically stressful environments with poor food and sleep deprivation. Our vote is for more education and to help people fall in love with their brains and take better care of them without substances that can harm them.

Another post that got a lot of attention was "Alcohol Is Not a Health Food." The constant messaging from the alcohol industry has people feeling they must drink two glasses of wine a day to be healthy. Yet, the evidence from our brain imaging studies is the exact opposite. Even a glass of beer or wine per day can be harmful to the brain and can make it look toxic. Alcohol contains carbohydrates that do not have any nutritional value. Alcohol is unique in that it contains 7 calories per gram instead of the typical 4 calories per gram found in other carbohydrates. Alcohol use is associated with fatty liver disease, peripheral neuropathies (pain and tingling in hands, legs, and feet), damage to neurons, especially those in the cerebellum, which is involved in physical and thought coordination and mood. It interferes with the absorption of vitamin B_1, which predisposes people to serious cognitive problems.

Alcohol decreases firing in the prefrontal cortex,[50] the most human and thoughtful part of the brain. It also disrupts sleep. In a 2015 study, people with a certain gene called *HTR2B* Q20*, found in 2.2 percent of the population, were more likely to have aggressive outbursts, get into

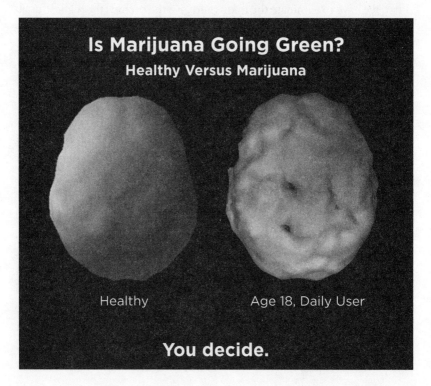

Is Marijuana Going Green?
Healthy Versus Marijuana

Healthy   Age 18, Daily User

You decide.

fights, and act rashly while drinking.[51] Even those who think of themselves as nice people when sober can turn into jerks when drunk. Another study found that nearly 25 percent of people surveyed said they became less agreeable, less responsible, and less intelligent when drinking alcohol compared to when they were sober.[52] Alcohol predisposes you to sugar abuse, stimulates your appetite, prolongs the time you sit during a meal, and is associated with continued eating even though you feel full. Alcohol exerts substantial influence on the circulation in your pancreas, increasing the production of insulin, which can lead to low blood sugar levels, which worsens your decisions.

And it gets worse. In 2015, the prestigious journal *Lancet* published a review of 115,000 subjects in which researchers found that alcohol decreased the risk of heart attacks, but increased the risk of cancer and physical injuries. High intake was associated with increased death from all causes.[53] Alcohol is also a known carcinogen and associated with 5.8 percent of all cancer deaths.[54]

Jürgen Rehm, director of the Social and Epidemiological Research Department at the Centre for Addiction and Mental Health in Toronto, Ontario, Canada, wrote, "Very simply, the cancers that have been determined

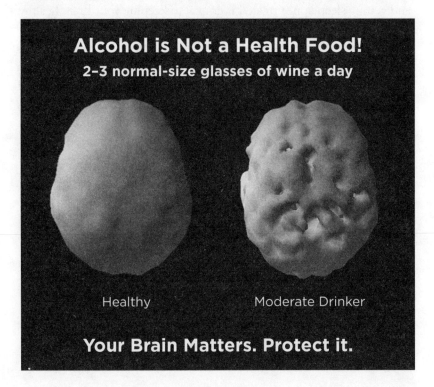

Alcohol is Not a Health Food!
2–3 normal-size glasses of wine a day

Healthy   Moderate Drinker

Your Brain Matters. Protect it.

previously to be caused by alcohol have been confirmed. There is no discussion about whether alcohol causes these cancers. The fact that alcohol is a carcinogen has been clearly confirmed." The cancers that Rehm refers to include those of the oral cavity, pharynx, larynx, esophagus, breast, colon, rectum, gallbladder, and liver.[55] There are other ways to decrease your risk of heart disease that do not increase your risk of cancer.

Less alcohol is better, and none is perfectly fine. You are not less of a man or a woman if you do not drink. You are not less mature, less interesting, or less fun as an adult if you do not drink. The good news is that your body can start to heal quickly if you stop drinking.[56]

Sleep Apnea

Another significant risk factor is sleep apnea, which includes loud snoring, stopped breathing at night, and chronic tiredness during the day. Sleep apnea is terrible for your health and your partner, who is also not getting a good night's sleep. Untreated sleep apnea triples your risk of dementia and depression and makes it hard to lose weight. Sleep apnea looks like early Alzheimer's disease on SPECT scans. Knowing whether you have it and getting sleep apnea treated is critical to keeping your brain healthy. Too many people find out they have sleep apnea, then never follow through with the treatment because they hate wearing the continuous positive airway pressure (CPAP) mask. Unfortunately, because the brain is so oxygen sensitive, untreated sleep apnea literally kills brain cells. If you are having trouble getting used to the CPAP, go back to the doctor as often as needed to get different strategies for treating this. There are a variety of CPAP masks available. Find one that works for you.

Insomnia

Insomnia can also hurt your brain. In fascinating new research, scientists have shown that your brain actually cleans or washes itself during sleep. The brain has a special waste management system that helps get rid of toxins that build up during the day, including the plaques thought to be responsible for Alzheimer's disease. During the day your brain is so busy managing your life that this cleaning system is pretty much turned off. Without healthy sleep, the cleaning crew does not have enough time to do their job and trash build ups, causing brain fog and memory prob-

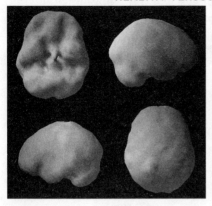 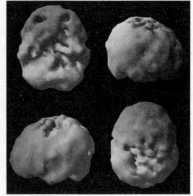

Healthy   Sleep Apnea

lems. How would your home look if no one cleaned for a month? That is the effect chronic insomnia can have on your brain.

In one study,

- Soldiers who got 7 hours of sleep at night were 98 percent accurate on the range.
- Those who got 6 hours of sleep were only 50 percent accurate.
- Those who got 5 hours of sleep were 28 percent accurate.
- Those who got 4 hours of sleep were only 15 percent accurate.

When you do not sleep, blood flow to your brain goes down and you are much more likely to make bad decisions. Focus on getting 7 to 8 hours of sleep every night. See Part 4 for more strategies on getting great sleep.

Excessive Stress

Excessive stress is another major risk factor for both depression and dementia. Some examples are these:

- Taking care of a loved one with a mental illness or a parent with dementia.
- Having a serious medical ailment like cancer.
- Losing a loved one, either through death or divorce.

Whenever you're exposed to a flood of stress hormones, it not only disrupts your sleep, but it can damage your immune system and actually shrink the memory centers in your brain. Because stress is everywhere, all of us would benefit from a regular stress management practice. Exercise and meditation can help, but our personal favorite is medical hypnosis, which Daniel has used with patients for many years.

Research has shown that medical hypnosis can calm your emotional brain and help you focus at the same time. It helps break addictions and treats depression, especially when it is combined with the ANT-killing technique we discuss in Part 4. It also helps with sleep.[57] See Part 4 for more strategies to bust up stress.

Untreated Depression, PTSD, and ADD/ADHD

Untreated depression doubles the risk of Alzheimer's disease in women and quadruples it in men. Some scientists think that depression in later life is actually the beginning of early Alzheimer's disease. Untreated PTSD also increases the risk of accelerated aging and Alzheimer's disease.

Untreated ADD or ADHD increases your risk for both depression and dementia. Studies have shown that ADD is associated with low activity in the prefrontal cortex, which, as mentioned before, acts as the brain's brake and stops you from saying or doing impulsive things. When the prefrontal cortex's activity is low, people tend to be easily distracted and have trouble controlling themselves, so it is very hard to stay on track and consistently make good decisions, even though that is their desire. In addition, ADD is associated with many of the other risk factors for dementia, including drug and alcohol abuse, smoking, traumatic brain injuries,[58] excessive stress, depression, and obesity. If you are disorganized or have a short attention span, get assessed and treated. It could save your brain. And it's never too late to get ADD treated. One of our favorite patients first came to see Daniel when she was ninety-four because she couldn't focus and could never finish reading the newspaper. A month after she started treatment—and with a big smile on her face—she told Daniel that she had read her first book.

Just because you have depression or ADD does not mean you have to take medicine to treat them. We are not opposed to medicine, but it is important to know that nutrition, exercise, omega-3s and other supplements, and learning to eliminate the automatic negative thoughts (if you also have depression) have also been found to be helpful in treating these disorders.

Lack of Exercise

If you exercise less than twice a week, you have an increased risk of dementia. You can eliminate that risk today by exercising more than twice a week. Physical exercise is the fountain of youth; it's critical to keeping your brain vibrant and young. If you want to attack Alzheimer's disease, depression, obesity, and aging all at once, move every day. In fact exercise is one of the most powerful antiaging tools, and it directly fights depression, anxiety, heart disease, diabetes and cancer. But be careful and don't overdo it. See Part 4 for more information on Brain Warrior physical exercise.

No New Learning and Addiction to Gadgets

No new learning or being addicted to your e-mail, text messages, or video games increases your risk of dementia and depression. In one study sponsored by Hewlett-Packard, people who were addicted to their gadgets lost ten IQ points over a year. It was more harmful than smoking marijuana, which also decreases IQ. You can decrease these risk factors today by limiting your gadgets and adding mental exercise to your life. See Part 4 for more information on new learning.

Standard American Diet

If you want to avoid depression and dementia you have to get your food right. The standard American diet, filled with sugar and pesticide-laden and processed foods, increases your risk of dementia and depression. In Part 3 we will give you a detailed nutrition plan to power your brain and body that decreases your risk for accelerated aging, depression, and dementia.

Increasing Age

Increasing age is the biggest risk factor for dementia. As we age we have less room for error. Daniel turned sixty-two this year and after looking at thousands of older brains, he knows he is in a war for the health of his brain. It is "normal," but not optimal or mandatory, to have your brain shrink with age; we want no part of it, and you should not just accept it as your fate.

If you have any of these risk factors, now is the time to get very serious about reversing these problems so that you can remain vibrant and sharp for as long as possible. You do not want to end up as a burden on your family.

BRAIN WARRIOR LESLIE

Leslie, who had the mother with Alzheimer's, took action and became a Brain Warrior. Her first scan showed really low overall activity. She was vulnerable to getting Alzheimer's. Rather than let the scan depress her, it motivated her, and she did everything we discussed, including adopting the Brain Warrior diet and a regular exercise program, improving her sleep, taking her supplements, and adding meditation into her life—among other lifestyle changes. A year later her brain was markedly improved, as were her sleep, mood, and memory. Plus she got her kids in the act. By being a healthy role model, she taught them to love their brains too. You are not stuck with the brain you have; you can make it better.

LESLIE'S BRAIN

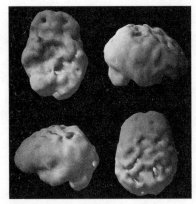
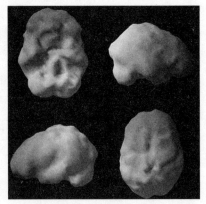

Before, Vulnerable

After, Healthier, Less Vulnerable

Brain Warrior Assessment Takeaways

Check the Brain Warrior Assessments you intend to complete over the next month.

❏ Assess your strategy for getting healthy.
  ▸ Develop brain envy.
  ▸ Avoid anything that hurts your brain.
  ▸ Engage in regular brain healthy habits.

❏ Assess your brain.
  ▸ Know your brain type (amenclinics.com).
  ▸ Take the Brain Fit WebNeuro test (mybrainfitlife.com).

❏ Know and optimize your important health numbers; don't just normalize them.
  ▸ BMI
  ▸ WHtR
  ▸ Blood pressure
  ▸ CBC
  ▸ General metabolic panel
  ▸ Fasting glucose
  ▸ Cholesterol panel
  ▸ HbA_{1c}
  ▸ Vitamin D
  ▸ Thyroid panel
  ▸ C-Reactive Protein
  ▸ Homocysteine
  ▸ Ferritin
  ▸ Testosterone
  ▸ Estrogen and progesterone in women

❏ Assess and fight the war strategically on multiple fronts.
  ▸ Blood flow
  ▸ Inflammation
  ▸ Gut health
  ▸ Blood sugar levels
  ▸ Antioxidant support
  ▸ Detoxification

- Nerve cell membrane fluidity
- Nutrient and amino acid loading

❏ Always assess where you are and engage in prevention strategies. The best way to prevent Alzheimer's and accelerated aging is to prevent all of the illnesses that are associated with them, such as:
  - Obesity, hypertension, heart disease, and diabetes
  - Low thyroid, estrogen, progesterone, and testosterone
  - Smoking and drug and alcohol abuse
  - Sleep apnea
  - Insomnia
  - Excessive stress
  - Untreated ADD, depression, and PTSD
  - Lack of exercise
  - Lack of new learning
  - Standard American diet

PART 3

Sustenance of a Brain Warrior

High-Powered Nutrition for a Victorious Life

Everyone has a doctor in him or her; we just have to help it in its work. The natural healing force within each one of us is the greatest force in getting well. Our food should be our medicine. Our medicine should be our food.

—HIPPOCRATES

TEN BRAIN WARRIOR NUTRITION PRINCIPLES

You cannot exercise, meditate, or supplement your way out of a bad diet. Food is medicine or it is poison. High-quality nutrition is one of the most important strategies for winning the war for the health of your brain and body. In any war, you must have a command center that has reliable information (food) to give clear orders to the troops (cells and organs). While the ball of gray matter between your ears weighs only about three pounds, it uses 20 to 30 percent of the calories you consume. It consumes more calories proportionally than any other part of your body and requires high-octane fuel to function at its peak. It's impossible to win the war if you feed the troops toxic, addictive, processed, pesticide-laden foods that damage your health. In fact, if you do, we wonder if you're working for the enemy—early death and destruction. When you eat poorly it's the equivalent of providing faulty intelligence to your command center. In turn, you incapacitate your elite forces. That's *self-sabotage*! With a little forethought, you can eat better than ever, while providing high-quality nutrition to your body to build and sustain your health.

There are mixed messages everywhere about what and how to eat for optimal health. While the intentions of the health food industry may be good, the messages are often contradictory and confusing. In fact, over the last two decades, the diet industry has become divided (and, as a result, divisive) between two schools of thought: *plants versus protein.*

We've seen people argue about vegetarian versus paleo diets more heatedly than others debate politics or religion! Each camp manages to root out just enough evidence to support its own position but rarely shows any evidence supporting the opposing view—because it has become about their philosophy, about *winning,* instead of about promoting health. The result has been nutritional chaos. You can be a vegetarian and be extremely unhealthy if you fill your body with pasta, bread, potatoes, and sugar. This was the case with one of our own physicians at

Amen Clinics who was surprised when he found out all of his important numbers were in the disease-promoting ranges. The same is true for paleo diets if you consume excessive protein (which creates oxidative stress) and limit your intake of health-promoting plants, replacing them with artificial foods. Look at the labels of many of the low-carb "healthy" packaged foods, and you will be horrified when you realize most of what you are eating is artificial. The answer lies not in the polar extremes of diet, but in a reasonable, science-based and highly nutritious path. The truth is that your body doesn't care about your food philosophy. It needs what it needs. We have no interest in changing your philosophy. Whether you're a caveman or a vegan, we can help you optimize your health with some simple rules outlined in this chapter.

USE ONLY HIGH-PREMIUM FUEL FOR SUCCESS

The Brain Warrior's Way is a plan that includes *both* an abundance of illness-fighting nutrients from whole, living plant foods *and* a portion of high-quality protein (plant or animal), with a mixture of healthy fat to keep the brain sharp and muscles and organs functioning at peak performance. Imagine a plate with a balance of vegetables, fruits, nuts, seeds, and healthy fish, meats, or plant proteins that give your body *everything* it needs. Eating a diet that's 70 percent plant-based foods and 30 percent high-quality protein, with healthy fat mixed in, restores energy, optimizes brain and hormone functioning, reduces the risk of disease, and produces dramatic weight loss as the side effect.

The most effective warriors have used food as medicine for centuries. They ate to win! It's astounding how conscious many warrior tribes have been throughout history, before they had the convenience of modern science, test tubes, or the Internet for information. Their knowledge of these principles was based purely on how they felt and how they performed. If they were strong and winning they knew their diet was working. If they were weak and losing, they stopped eating whatever it was that was impairing their strength or mental function.

It's primarily in modern times that common sense has left the dinner table of warriors. One of our closest friends, Lieutenant Colonel Daniel Johnston, past medical director of the U.S. Army's Comprehensive Soldier and Family Fitness program, told us that our servicemen and -women were offered unlimited Baskin-Robbins ice cream during lunch and dinner—completely insane.

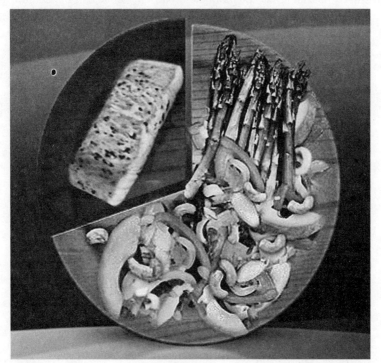

ANCIENT WARRIORS ATE TO WIN

Spartans: Spartans were arguably the most elite ancient warriors. From the age of seven, life for a Spartan was focused on a warrior culture. Victory was the most important thing. Food was simply a *necessity*, a *tool* used to increase strength. Spartans often practiced hunger in preparation for battle when food would not be available. Spartans were passionate about fitness and considered *any* unhealthy habits weakness. Bread was eaten on *occasion*. The Spartan diet primarily focused on meat, fish, sheep, goat milk, and black broth (boiled pig legs, blood, salt, and vinegar). Even Spartan wine was watered down to avoid intoxication. Any form of overindulgence, which dulled the wits or diminished strength, was frowned upon. Spartans were serious about winning!

Sarmatians: Rumored to be the offspring of Amazon women and Scythian men, the Sarmatians were revered female warriors who

(CONTINUED)

lived near the Black Sea and ate a nutrient-dense diet of seafood, vegetables, fermented milk, and wild game. Hippocrates wrote this about this ferocious group of women:

> Their women, so long as they are virgins, ride, shoot, throw
> the javelin while mounted, and fight with their enemies. . . .
> They have no right breast; for while they are yet babies their
> mothers make red-hot a bronze instrument constructed for
> this very purpose and apply it to the right breast and cauterize
> it, so that its growth is arrested, and all its strength and bulk
> are diverted to the right shoulder and right arm.

These women were rumored to be extraordinarily strong and healthy. If they could survive having a breast removed and the likely infection that would follow, they were seen as having almost super-human strength. While it's uncertain if these formidable women are historical fact or myth, ancient writings and statues depict female warriors proudly showing off their breastless chests. Fact or not, Tana has adopted a similar attitude (shirt on) and diet.

Ninjas: The Ninjas believed that food and medicine were of the same roots and for the same purpose. These petite, lean warriors couldn't weigh more than about 140 pounds due to the acrobatic nature of their art and the need to be "invisible" and *really fast.* If you're a vegetarian you'll appreciate the diet of these stealthy war-riors. They tended to avoid meat because they believed it dulled the senses. They obtained some protein from quail eggs and soybeans. They had a heavily plant-based diet, avoiding foods that added ex-cess body weight (including bulky muscle), bad breath, or body odor. In emergencies, Ninjas would eat frogs, snakes, bugs, dirt, and just about any nonpoisonous plant. On the road, Ninjas ate pow-er-packed, medicinal-type dumplings made of licorice, mint, starch, other local herbs (ailment specific), and plums. Ninjas relied heavily on herbal medicine and often included it in their food.

Samurai: A traditional prewar meal for the Samurai often con-sisted of chestnuts, kelp, and abalone. The Samurai warrior believed that success would be achieved through nourishing the mind, body, and spirit equally. The Samurai warriors, notably remembered for their "indomitable spirit," commitment to action, mastery over fear, and total focus, lived by an ethical code called *Bushido* (the way of the warrior). In addition to undergoing the intensely brutal physical training, they were equally dedicated to education, arts, and meditation. In fact their motto was "The pen and the sword in accord." It's believed that much of their success in battle could be attributed to the daily practice of meditation and self-hypnosis. Their native country, Japan, offered a great variety of fruit, vegetables, seaweed, and seafood for these revered warriors to consume.

Mongols: The Mongols are often referred to as Tartars, thought to be the inventors of steak tartar. Mongolian warriors were some of the most savage warriors ever known. Because it was nearly impossible for these nomads to farm, the Mongolian warrior subsisted primarily on fermented milk products and meat. Troops often had to travel for weeks in harsh terrain, without starting a fire to avoid being detected. As a result, their diet consisted of nutrient-dense dried meat. They would scavenge wild onions, berries, and greens they saw along the way when possible. They rode mares and milked them. They ate the raw meat of their horses, and were known to place the meat under their saddles, allowing it to mix with sweat, which tenderized it. In emergencies they would cut the arteries of a horse and drink its blood.

Mongolian warriors were notoriously strong, with thick bones and healthy teeth. They could go days without eating when necessary and still stay strong. It's believed Mongolian strength and endurance resulted from their diet. This is in stark contrast to many of their enemies, such as the Jurchens, who ate a primarily vegetable- and grain-based diet. The Jurchens were weaker and smaller in stature and suffered from tooth decay.

Vikings: Vikings enjoyed an incredibly diverse diet compared to other cultures, including wild game, seafood, greens, roots, berries, nuts, seeds, sourdough bread, and many forms of fermented foods. These deadly warriors were often depicted by their enemies as being the "perfect human specimens" due to their relatively large size and fair features. It's true that Viking warriors and noblemen were taller and more muscular than most of the enemies they encountered. However, commoners and slaves were actually quite unhealthy. The lower classes and slaves were uneducated about food preparation, and lacked the same diversity in their diets.

(CONTINUED)

Apaches: The legendary Apache warriors are often referred to as the "Ninjas of the Americas." Apaches were conscious about what the animals they ate had eaten. As hunter-gatherers, Apaches ate nuts, berries, vegetables, and some *clean* meat. They hunted deer, rabbit, mule, and other vegetarian animals. They refused to eat fish, "squirmy creatures," or any animal that ate other animals or squirmy creatures. While they valued protein in their diet, they would forgo meat before they would eat an unclean source because they believed that they themselves consumed all the things that the animals they ate had consumed. They were a strong, muscular, fierce, and strategic-thinking people who were capable of enduring relentless hardship.

Roman Legion Soldiers: Clearly the largest and wealthiest military force of its time, the Roman Legion was also one of the few ancient armies known to eat a primarily plant- and grain-based diet, especially during battle when they traveled long distances with road rations. Roman warriors were known for their tough military training and endurance. However, a large part of their success can be attributed to the sheer size of their army. The booming Roman economy and temperate climate afforded a wide variety of fruits and vegetables to the wealthy, but not to the commoners, who often died of starvation and disease associated with large population growth. Many men joined the army to avoid starvation and dire living conditions. Unfortunately, soldiers weren't immune to the rampant disease running through the cities they policed. One of the strengths of the Roman Legion during war was their practice of cyclically sending soldiers to battle in waves to ensure an ever-ready front line. As the front lines became fatigued and dehydrated, they moved to the back to rest and rehydrate.

Gladiators: By design, gladiators ate a high-carbohydrate diet of fruit, vegetables, legumes, and grains. Commonly referred to as "barley men," this unique subset of warrior wanted to be bulky! Gladiators, chosen to entertain audiences (sometimes by enslavement, sometimes by choice), can be likened to some modern-day professional athletes. Often considered the workingman's hero, gladiators inspired hope in the lower classes, who chanted for them in the arena and drew likenesses of them on building walls.

In spite of the reverence bestowed on them, life as a gladiator was brutal and usually short. They were strong and muscular, but they also wanted an extra layer of fat to keep vital organs and arteries from being slashed so they could continue fighting. It made for a good spectacle to have bleeding gashes that were not fatal. They trained for strength and explosiveness to survive an intense, life-threatening fight that could last ten to fifteen minutes. They didn't need the long-term endurance of a marathoner. They rarely lived past the age of thirty. Let us repeat: *Gladiators ate a (high-quality) high-carbohydrate/low-protein diet because they wanted and needed to be bulky and have explosive, short-term energy.*

Even though we do not recommend all of the ancient warrior foods, especially the black broth of the Spartans, the point is clear: Warriors eat to win. Their diets matter to their ability to survive and thrive. Yours does too.

Once you commit to being a Brain Warrior you will quickly notice that you have more energy, better focus, a better memory, better moods, and even a flatter tummy within a matter of weeks. A number of new studies have reported that a healthful diet, like ours, is associated with significantly lower risks of Alzheimer's disease and depression.[59] Plus, when you decide to take that first step and eat healthfully, your cravings will start to settle down quickly. It will be the beginning of a new, healthy relationship with food.

Don't worry if you're just starting out and can't cook. Tana literally couldn't cook *at all* when she met Daniel eleven years ago. Daniel often says that Tana went from "disaster to master" in the kitchen. Contrary to popular belief, it's not because Tana loves to cook. She doesn't! It's because she loves to *serve!* She wants to serve our family and keep us healthy. Preparing healthy food is one of the most important ways she does it. Believe us, if she can do it and make it simple, you can, too!

Contrary to what most people think, eating in a brain healthy way is not more expensive; it is less expensive. Tana knows firsthand how expensive it is to be sick, to drop out of school, and to quit her job. What has choosing an unhealthy lifestyle cost *you*? The exciting news is that you can start feeling better quickly. Your medical bills will be lower and your productivity will go way up. And what price can you put on feeling amazing?

The Brain Warrior Nutrition Principles are very simple and designed to guide you through the rest of your life. There are no gimmicks, no designer foods to buy, and no radical calorie cutting. We know you won't do any program that is complicated or requires you to eat boring foods for the next twenty years. Brain Warrior food is delicious, energizing, and healing.

THE NUTRITION PRINCIPLES: DAILY FUEL FOR ULTIMATE VICTORY

If you are going to eat right to think right, it is critical to make sure your food is loaded with proper nutrients that your body is able to effectively digest and absorb. Here are ten simple principles.

Principle 1:

Focus on High-Quality Calories

There is no such thing as "empty calories." The term *junk food* is an oxymoron. It's either junk that is driving you toward illness or food that is medicine for your brain and body!

The quality of your food matters significantly more than the quantity of it for getting healthy, losing weight, or preventing illness. Compare a 500-calorie cinnamon roll to a 500-calorie plate of salmon, spinach, red bell peppers, blueberries, and walnuts. One will drain your energy and increase inflammation; the other will supercharge your mind and decrease your risk of accelerated aging. Plus one meal is gobbled quickly, spiking your blood sugar and doing a hit-and-run on pleasure centers, while the other is consumed more slowly and will help you feel fuller, happier, and more stable for longer.

Getting healthy is not as simple as calories in versus calories out—some calories hijack your hormones, taste buds, and health. Eating sugar and processed food, even in small amounts, increases cravings, stress hormones, and promotes illness. You can actually eat much more if you eat high-quality food that gives you energy and turns on the hormones of metabolism, as outlined in these rules.

Bebac and Mokolo, two male western lowland gorillas, live at the Cleveland Metroparks Zoo. When Bebac and Mokolo were barely middle age (about their mid-twenties); they were overweight and had developed heart disease. They also demonstrated abnormal behaviors, such as regurgitating and re-eating their food and pulling out their hair and eating it. These behaviors are unheard of in wild gorillas.

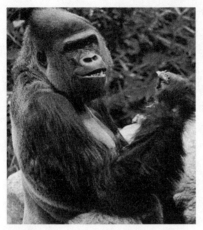

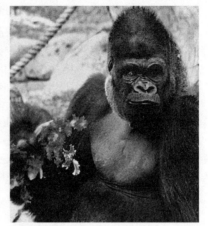

Bebac

Mokolo

In the wild, gorillas usually die from things like acute illnesses, such as infections, or human poaching. Chronic diseases, such as heart disease and diabetes, are rare in gorillas living freely in the tropical forests of sub-Saharan Africa. So why is *heart disease* the number one cause of death among captive gorillas? This discrepancy has perplexed veterinarians for years.

The veterinarians at the Cleveland zoo became concerned about Bebac and Mokolo and decided to analyze all the aspects of their lives. They quickly zeroed in on the gorillas' diet as the culprit. Sadly, the diet for most captive gorillas resembles the standard American diet. Instead of dozens of pounds of wild greens, fiber, berries, nuts and seeds, and high-quality protein from bugs naturally ingested in the wild, captive gorillas are commonly fed "nutritional cookies" made from grains, sugar, and starch. The intention may be well meaning, as a way to ensure the gorillas get all their vitamins, minerals and amino acids, yet it completely misses the mark. This reminds us of children's vitamins loaded with sugar and artificial coloring—yet another weapon of mass destruction!

Things changed at the zoo when the veterinarians decided to replace the cookies with a more wholesome diet of vegetables, fruits, and leafy greens such as dandelion greens, romaine, green beans, endive, berries, flax, bamboo, and alfalfa hay. In addition to the new diet, the gorillas were required to be more active. Zookeepers scattered the food throughout their habitat, ensuring they would have to forage for their meals rather than being presented with cookies they could gobble up quickly (fast food was out). Instead of spending a few minutes munching cookies, the gorillas began to spend up to 75 percent of their day foraging and eating—about the same amount of time they would forage in the wild.

Although the wild diet was nearly double the calories of the processed cookies, the gorillas lost weight. In one year, the gorillas, who initially weighed 430 and 460 pounds, each lost about 65 pounds. And tests showed improvement in heart function for Bebac and the slowing of progression of heart disease for Mokolo. Amazingly, the neurotic behavior of regurgitating and re-eating their food also stopped. Researchers aren't sure if the gorillas did this because the cookies upset their stomach, or worse, they may have regurgitated their food because they wanted to taste the sugar in the cookies again and again (their pleasure centers went wild). Hair-plucking behaviors also became a rare occurrence.

Thinking of the dramatic change in the gorillas is cause for us to consider some of the patients we have worked with who suffer from similar behaviors (uncontrolled hair pulling and regurgitating food). It makes us wonder if the gorillas were really neurotic or if they were being poisoned by an unnatural diet of processed food, grains, sugar, and starch. Similar to the gorillas, humans have been demonstrating an increase in chronic diseases and certain unnatural behaviors as the intake of processed food has increased. At Amen Clinics, we put nutrition at the center of our treatment plans. The patients who take their nutrition seriously get dramatically better results than those who don't.

One more interesting note: veterinarians noticed that Bebac and Mokolo were grumpy for about a week after having the sugar-filled cookies removed from their diets. But just like the people we coach, they soon got over it, lost their cravings, and got healthy. A week of crabbiness seems like a minor inconvenience to have a healthier heart and decreased neurotic behaviors. In other words, lovingly discipline your spoiled, petulant inner child the same way you would your own children when they want to do something harmful or dangerous.

■

Read the labels of everything you buy and understand them. Be serious about high-quality nutrition.

■

Principle 2:

Drink Plenty of Water

Your brain is 80 percent water. Keeping your brain hydrated helps optimize the brain's power and prevent dehydration. Did you know that by simply hydrating you will increase your physical strength and power by 19 percent! If you are an athlete, this is a critical point. You'll also make muscle gains more rapidly and have improved aerobic function and endurance. That means the opposite is also true; you will be weaker and have less endurance if you are dehydrated.

Being dehydrated by just 2 percent impairs performance in tasks that require attention, immediate memory skills, and physical performance.[60] It is also associated with brain atrophy (shrinkage), poor concentration, memory difficulties, diminished school performance, and increased sensitivity to pain.[61] Children who are dehydrated have more problems in school.[62] A research study found that pilots who were dehydrated had poorer performance in the cockpit, especially as it related to working memory, spatial orientation, and cognitive performance.[63]

We recommend drinking half your body weight in ounces—for example, if you weigh 160 pounds, drink 80 ounces of water daily. If you are obese consult a physician about consuming more than 120 ounces a day, as you must be sure not to cause an electrolyte imbalance. When losing weight, your body needs water to flush out the toxins that are released by stored body fat. Staying hydrated also helps prevent overeating. Oftentimes when people think they're hungry, they're actually thirsty. Drinking 16 ounces of water 30 minutes before a meal or snack helps you eat less and still feel satiated. However, avoid drinking water with your meal, as it slows down digestion by diluting stomach acid.

Replace sugary drinks with water. Just cutting out sugary drinks and fruit juice cuts an average of 400 calories per day from the typical American diet! That's either a lot more healthy food you will get to eat instead or a lot of calories you will be losing if you need to lose weight (actually it equates to losing 40 pounds a year, if you do not replace those calories)!

Be deliberate about your water intake and limit anything that dehydrates you (caffeine, alcohol, and diuretics). When you sweat through exercise, make sure to rehydrate. Tana starts the day with 16 ounces of warm water with freshly squeezed lemon and fresh ginger, which is cleansing and alkalinizing.

Daniel doesn't really like drinking water, which is why he starts his day with one of Tana's smoothie recipes, which has 20 ounces of water. He also created Brain Boost on the Go, the Think Drink, which contains L-theanine from green tea, vitamins B_6 and B_{12}, folate, and an organic fruit blend of acai, goji, mangosteen and noni, to encourage his water consumption throughout the day. When Daniel just carries a bottle of water with him, he rarely drinks it, but if he pours Brain Boost on the Go into the water, it will all be gone quickly. Another strategy we use is drinking sparkling water with a little bit of SweetLeaf chocolate stevia. It is heaven for those of us with a bit of a sweet tooth, without any of the toxicity of sugar or artificial sweeteners. Remember, there is no suffering for Brain Warriors.

■

Focus on drinking water daily.

■

Principle 3:

Eat High-Quality Protein in Small Doses Throughout the Day

Protein plays a major role in the healthy growth and functioning of your cells, tissues, and organs. Other than water, protein is the most abundant substance in your body. We think of protein as medicine that should be taken in small doses at least every 4 to 5 hours, with every meal and snack.

Consuming protein helps balance the hormones of metabolism required to stave off hunger. It also triggers your body to release the hormone pancreatic peptide YY (PYY), which improves sensitivity to the hormone leptin. Leptin tells your brain when you're full and to stop eating. Protein also stimulates the release of glucagon, which stabilizes blood sugar and prevents energy crashes—the opposite of what insulin does. After eating a protein-containing meal or snack, you feel fuller longer and burn more calories than you do after eating high-carb, sugar-filled foods. Think of insulin like a selfish hoarder: it wants to hold on to fat, and it is stimulated most quickly by sugar and simple carbs. Think of glucagon as a philanthropist that wants to give everything away. Glucagon wants to use up energy and fat. It is released most easily when you consume protein.

Protein also provides your body with amino acids. Your muscles, skin, hair, many hormones, neurotransmitters, and other body parts all need a reliable and regular intake of essential amino acids for optimal health. Your body can produce *some* of the amino acids it needs, but not all of them—those that can't be manufactured in your body must come from food. These are called essential amino acids. They must be included in your diet on a regular basis, because your body can't store them for future use. Plant foods such as nuts, seeds, legumes, and some grains and vegetables contain only some of the twenty amino acids we need. Fish, poultry, and most meats contain all of them. The same is true for essential fatty acids, which your body also requires but can't produce on its own.

TOO MUCH OF A GOOD THING

In the case of protein more is not better (which is why we want you to think of having it in small doses)! Small amounts of high-quality protein are crucial to good health. But too much protein, or choosing poor-quality protein, can actually be detrimental to your health. Our bodies are simply not designed to effectively process large quantities of protein at one time. Eating too much protein causes increased oxidative stress and inflammation in the body. This contributes to accelerated aging, inefficient DNA repair, and disease. For some people it can be hard on the kidneys and liver as well. These organs are responsible for detoxification and elimination of waste products created by protein metabolism, which can become a burden if there is an excess.

Quality is more important than quantity. High-quality animal protein is more expensive than industrially raised animal protein. Unfortunately, people who make animal protein the foundation of their diet often sacrifice quality to make up for quantity. Rather than choosing the highest-quality meat, many turn to processed and cured meat, which often contains excessive amounts of salt, sugar, and fake fillers. Also, industrially raised meat is about 30 percent higher than grass-fed meat in palmitic acid (a type of unhealthy saturated fat), which is associated with cardiovascular disease.

One of our biggest concerns with a high-protein diet is that if you overcrowd your diet with protein, you don't make enough space on your plate for the energy-giving, disease-preventing nutrients that come from whole, living plant foods. Balance is critical for Brain Warriors to thrive for the long term, which is why thinking of 70 percent plant-based foods and 30 percent protein is so important.

SHAKE HANDS WITH PROTEIN

Because most people don't carry food scales everywhere they go or have nutritional information available, a simple strategy to figure out how much protein to eat is to use the palm of your hand as a size guide. If you "shake hands" with protein, you'll get just what you need.

■

Take protein like medicine at every meal to help keep your blood sugar balanced, so you make good decisions throughout the day.

■

Principle 4:

Eat Smart Carbohydrates
(Low Glycemic, High Fiber)

The fastest way to lower insulin levels, balance blood sugar, decrease cravings, and jump-start weight loss is to decrease the amount of high-glycemic, low-fiber carbohydrates you eat. Focus on smart carbohydrates, which we define as low glycemic, meaning they do not quickly raise your blood sugar levels, while being high in fiber, such as those found in nonstarchy vegetables and lower glycemic fruits like blueberries, pears, and apples.

Getting the hormone insulin under control is critical to your overall mental and physical health. Insulin, made in the pancreas, is involved with how your body directs and uses its calories. Soon after you start eating, insulin increases and acts as a traffic cop to direct calories from carbohydrates, proteins, and fats into body tissues for immediate use or storage. A few hours later when insulin levels drop, the stored calories reenter your bloodstream and are used by your brain and body for fuel in between meals. Harvard endocrinologist and obesity expert David Ludwig calls insulin the "ultimate fat fertilizer."[64] Rats given insulin developed low blood sugar, ate more food, and gained more weight than rats not given insulin. Even when food was restricted, they still became fatter.[65] Insulin encourages fat cells to increase in both size and number. What drives the pancreas to increase insulin? Fast-digesting carbohydrates, especially sugar, refined grains, potato products, rice flour, many packaged gluten-free foods, and other high-glycemic foods that quickly turn to sugar.

Ludwig writes, "Overeating hasn't made our fat cells grow; our fat cells have been programmed to grow, and that has made us overeat!"

High insulin levels cause fat cells to hoard excessive amounts of glucose and fat. Insulin causes calories to go into fat cells but restricts them from coming out, so you feel endlessly hungry, even with plenty of fat on your body. Your energy becomes trapped inside your fat cells and your brain screams for help; stress hormones surge when blood sugar levels are low, so you feel like you have to eat more. It's a sadistic trap with a simple solution: Focus your diet on foods that lower insulin levels, such as healthy proteins, fats, and smart carbohydrates. Most people think of obesity as a condition of too many calories, but it is actually a condition of too few of the right kind. You can actually starve yourself fat!

THE GLYCEMIC INDEX AND GLYCEMIC LOAD

Get to know the glycemic index (GI) and glycemic load (GL) for the foods you eat. The GI rates carbohydrates according to their effects on blood sugar from a 50-gram load. It is ranked on a scale from one to 100+ (glucose is 100) with the low GI foods having a lower number (which means they do not spike your blood sugar, so they tend to be healthier) and the higher GI foods having a high number (which means they quickly elevate your blood sugar, so they are generally not as healthful). In general, we like to stay with foods that have a glycemic index value under 60. Research on the GI yielded some big surprises. For example, potatoes and bread were higher on the GI scale than either honey or table sugar!

GL is a more valuable indicator. GI doesn't take portion sizes into account. For example, watermelon has a high GI (72), but a low GL

(3.6). You have to eat a lot to raise your blood sugar. GL takes size, portion, and blood sugar into account all at once.

Eating a diet that is filled with low-glycemic foods will lower your blood glucose levels, decrease cravings, and help you focus. The table below shows the glycemic load for some common foods. Just because a food has a low GL does *not* necessarily mean it is good for you. For example, fructose has a low GL, but it is associated with hypertension and obesity because of how it is processed in the liver. Milk has a low GL, but comes from animals that were given antibiotics and hormones. The foods in the Brain Warrior's Way need to meet all of the ten rules to be considered healthful.

GLYCEMIC LOAD OF CARBOHYDRATE-CONTAINING FOODS

(Adapted and reprinted from *Always Hungry?* with permission)

FOOD GROUP	LOW (MOST FREE)	MODERATE (LIMIT)	HIGH (AVOID)
VEGETABLES			
	Alfalfa sprouts	Acorn squash	Boiled potatoes
	Artichokes	Beets	French fries
	Asparagus	Butternut squash	White potatoes
	Bamboo shoots	Green peas	
	Bean sprouts	Parsnips	
	Bok choy	Pumpkin	
	Broccoli	Sweet potatoes	
	Brussels sprouts	Yams	
	Cabbage		
	Carrots		
	Cauliflower		
	Celery		
	Chard/Swiss chard		
	Collard/mustard greens		
	Cucumbers		
	Green beans		

FOOD GROUP	LOW (MOST FREE)	MODERATE (LIMIT)	HIGH (AVOID)
	Kale		
	Leeks		
	Lettuces		
	Mushrooms		
	Okra		
	Onions		
	Peppers		
	Radishes		
	Snow peas		
	Spinach		
	Summer squash		
	Turnips		
	Water chestnuts		
	Zucchini		
FRUITS			
	Apples	Bananas	Dates
	Apricots	Cantaloupe	Dried fruit
	Avocados	Honeydew	Fruit juices and drinks
	Berries	Mango	Raisins
	Cherries	Papaya	
	Grapes	Pineapple	
	Grapefruit	Watermelon	
	Kiwi		
	Lemons		
	Limes		
	Nectarines		
	Oranges		
	Peaches		

(TABLE CONTINUES)

FOOD GROUP	LOW (MOST FREE)	MODERATE (LIMIT)	HIGH (AVOID)
	Pears		
	Plums		
	Tangerines		
	Tomatoes		
LEGUMES			
	Beans (all kinds except baked)	Peanut butter, sugar sweetened	
	Black-eyed peas		
	Chickpeas		
	Hummus		
	Lentils		
	Peanuts		
	Split peas		
NUTS			
	Almonds		
	Brazil nuts		
	Cashews		
	Hazelnuts		
	Nut butters, no added sugar		
	Pecans		
	Pistachios		
	Walnuts		
SEEDS			
	Chia		
	Pumpkin		
	Sesame		
	Sunflower		
DAIRY			
	Cheese	Milk	

FOOD GROUP	LOW (MOST FREE)	MODERATE (LIMIT)	HIGH (AVOID)
	Yogurt, no added sugar	Yogurt, sugar sweetened	
GRAINS			
		Amaranth	Bread, highly processed, including bagels, buns, corn bread, English muffins, pitas, rolls, and white and most wheat breads
		Barley	Breakfast cereals, low fiber
		Bread, minimally processed, including whole kernel, sprouted grain, and stone ground	Couscous
		Breakfast cereal, high fiber	Crackers
		Brown rice	Pancakes
		Buckwheat	Pasta
		Corn	Pizza
		Farro	Popcorn
		Oats	Pretzels
		Quinoa	Rice cakes
		Rye	Stuffing
		Wheat berries	Taco shell
		Wild rice	Tortilla
			Waffle
			White rice
DESSERTS, SWEETS, TREATS			
	Dark chocolate	Ice cream	Brownies
		Milk chocolate	Cake
			Candy

(TABLE CONTINUES)

FOOD GROUP	LOW (MOST FREE)	MODERATE (LIMIT)	HIGH (AVOID)
			Chips
			Cookies
			Custards
			Doughnuts
			Fruit roll-ups
			Pies
			Sorbet
SWEETENERS			
	Fructose (but goes to liver, avoid)	Honey	Glucose
	Agave (but goes to liver, avoid)	Table sugar	
	Erythritol		
	Stevia		

FIBER: THE SPECIAL CARBOHYDRATE

Fiber is a special type of carbohydrate. It differs from simple carbohydrates because it can't be digested by humans. But it's very important because it plays an active role in optimizing your health. Unfortunately, the average American consumes less than 15 grams of fiber daily, which is dangerously low. Women should consume 25 to 30 grams of fiber daily, and men should strive to consume 30 to 38 grams.

Dietary fiber helps improve bowel function, reduces the risk of colon cancer, and helps stabilize blood sugar. High-fiber foods—such as broccoli, berries, onions, flaxseeds, nuts, green beans, cauliflower, celery, and sweet potatoes (the skin of one sweet potato has more fiber than a bowl of oatmeal!)—make you feel full faster and longer.

Fiber impacts digestion, starting from your first bite. High-fiber foods generally require longer chewing time, which slows down your eating. This gives the hormones of satiety time to communicate with your brain. In the stomach, fiber absorbs water and creates bulk, which can increase the time it takes for food to move out of the stomach. As a result, you'll feel full longer and be less likely to experience the rapid spikes in blood sugar that occur when food digests quickly and glucose is dumped into the blood. In the small intestines and all the way through to the colon, fiber keeps things moving while providing bulk. It's also where the fermentation process begins (a vital process for gut health). Both soluble and insoluble fiber are important in this process. Fast food is often very low in fiber by design. That way you eat it quickly and they can serve more people in the restaurants in less time.

Soluble fiber (found in foods such as apples, berries, flaxseeds, and supplements) provides food (prebiotics) to the friendly health-boosting bacteria in your gut. Digestive health is improved when the friendly bacteria are well fed and able to crowd out the bad bacteria that cause disease and reduce immunity. Friendly bacteria are also responsible for making certain vitamins, such as vitamin K and some B vitamins, and boosting immunity.

Insoluble fiber doesn't provide much benefit in the way of fermentation, but it does work like a broom, helping keep the intestines cleaned out. It also makes sure that the vital fermented products of the soluble fiber get distributed throughout the entire colon.

FIBER: WHAT IT CAN DO FOR YOU

- Decrease ghrelin—the hormone that tells you to eat more
- Help you feel full faster and longer
- Slow absorption of food
- Reduce LDL cholesterol
- Keep your digestive tract moving
- Reduce high blood pressure
- Reduce the risk of cancer

Have 25–35 grams per day

The Brain Warrior's Way program places high importance on vegetable intake, which significantly increases both soluble and insoluble fiber. Even so, we believe it's still worthwhile to add fiber supplements to a morning smoothie or afternoon glass of water, especially in the beginning. This is especially helpful if you are insulin resistant or have high cholesterol. Short-chain fatty acids, which are responsible for regulating cholesterol and insulin responses, are made in the colon, so keeping it healthy is critical to proper metabolic function.

Principle 5:

Focus Your Diet on Healthy Fats

About 60 percent of the solid weight of your brain is fat. Fat is not the enemy. Good fats are essential to your health. In a study from the Mayo Clinic, people who ate a fat-based diet had a 42 percent lower risk of developing Alzheimer's disease, while people who ate a carbohydrate-based diet (think rice, potatoes, and pasta) were four times more likely to develop the disease. People who ate a protein-based diet had a 21 percent lower risk of developing Alzheimer's disease.[66]

When the American Heart Association launched a campaign to reduce saturated fat in the standard American diet, what the public heard was that they should cut out as much fat as possible. Unfortunately, this led to people also restricting essential fatty acids (which are called essential for a reason) from their diets—not just saturated fat, but all fat. Fat was demonized as the cause of heart disease and many other health problems.

The food advertisers saw a plump opportunity and jumped on it. The fat-free craze was born! Americans began a free-for-all; gorging on highly processed, fat-free carbohydrates—fat-free cookies and cakes, bagels, crackers, and more. And why not? Carbohydrates wouldn't make us fat, the experts said—only fat could make us fat! Of course, no one actually bothered to check all this out before presenting it as fact, and it backfired in a big fat way. During the war against fat, Americans indulged in fat-free, chemical-laden, processed food. And, while the fat-free witch hunt continued, they consumed more carbohydrates, sugar, and calories than ever before. This triggered an obesity epidemic that is still going strong. Since the early 1980s, obesity rates in the United States rose from 12 percent to an astonishing 36 percent in 2015. There was also an increase in sudden cardiac arrest (heart attacks), diabetes, hypertension, cancer, depression, and dementia among people who were unknowingly starving their bodies of essential fatty acids in an attempt to eradicate fat from their diets. Without healthy fat our bodies can't effectively use fat-soluble vitamins such as A, D, E, and K. Fats also play an important part in the health of brain function, cellular communication, production of important hormones, skin, hair, body temperature, and weight maintenance!

Eat more fat, lose more fat. It sounds contradictory, but science shows that it's true. In 2000, researchers in Boston analyzed two groups of people—one group on a low-fat diet (20 percent of calories from fat), the other group on a moderate-fat diet (35 percent of calories from fat). After eighteen months, people eating moderate amounts of fat lost a mean of 9 pounds and trimmed 2.7 inches from their waistlines. The low-fat group, however, *gained* a mean of 6.4 pounds and *added* 1 inch around the middle. What we find intriguing about this study is that more than half of the moderate-fat dieters were able to stick with the program for the entire eighteen months. Compare that to 80 percent of the low-fat dieters who found it too hard to stick with the program and dropped out. Healthy fats help with satiety. The key to boosting fat consumption for weight loss is eating healthy fats.

THE SKINNY ON FAT

While it's important to avoid fried fats, trans fats, and some saturated fats, cutting way back on healthy fats is harmful, because your body needs them for many crucial functions. Like protein, healthy fats stimulate the release of the hormone PYY, which helps you feel full. Your body also uses healthy fats to store energy, build healthy cells, support proper brain function, prevent oxidative damage and degenerative nerve disorders, and manufacture hormones. Fat is also *required* for your body to absorb and store certain vitamins, minerals, and nutrients (which is why it's a good idea to take nutritional supplements with a meal containing a little healthy fat). And you need a substantial amount of healthy fats (especially omega-3 fatty acids) in your diet (at regular intervals) to prevent the loss of your hard-earned muscles during weight loss.

Like with so many important topics in the world of optimal nutrition, the enthusiasm for fat-free eating was vastly oversimplified. Let's step back a bit and look at how different kinds of fats impact our health. As with carbohydrates, there are *good* fats and *bad* fats.

Omega-3 Fatty Acids

The family of omega-3 fatty acids is definitely good. These fats are crucial for optimal health and are called spring fats, for the vitality and energy they bring. Your brain needs specific types of essential omega-3 fatty acids, such as docosahexaenoic acid (DHA) and eicosapentaenoic acid (EPA), to function well. These omega-3 fatty acids are found in fish, such as salmon and tuna. Deficiencies in these vital fatty acids have been shown to be associated with age-related cognitive decline, psychological disturbances, depression, mood swings, and neuropathy (tingling in hands and feet). Similarly, these critical fatty acids are necessary for optimal immune response and improving cardiovascular health, joint health, skin quality, vision, and wound healing. Omega-3 fatty acids are especially important for pregnant women because they contribute to the development of a baby's eyes, brain, and immune system.

Eating fish benefits cognitive performance. A study from Swedish researchers that surveyed nearly five thousand fifteen-year-old boys found that those who ate fish more than once a week scored higher on standard intelligence tests than teens who ate no fish. A follow-up study found that teens eating fish more than once a week also had better grades at school than students with lower fish consumption. Other benefits of omega-3 fatty acids include improving attention in people with ADD and reducing the risk for psychosis.

Omega-6 Fatty Acids

Although omega-6 fatty acids are necessary, they can be harmful when you eat them in excess, so they're good *and* bad. Omega-6 fatty acids are found in most vegetable oils (soybean, sunflower, safflower, corn, and canola), as well as in many fried foods, cereals, and whole-grain breads. One of the benefits is that omega-6 fatty acids contribute to muscle health. However, eating too much of these fats is a problem because they cancel out the benefits of omega-3 fatty acids when the ratio of omega-6 to omega-3 is too high. The optimal ratio is less than 4 to 1 (omega-6 to omega-3). Most people who eat the standard American diet, which contains high levels of omega-6-rich vegetable oils, have an appalling ratio of up to 20 to 1 or higher. Translated into health terms, this is an inflammatory process at work in your body, putting you at risk for heart disease, cancer, diabetes, and a host of other health problems. A proper ratio of omega-6 fatty acids to omega-3 fatty acids has also been shown to decrease triglycerides and help prevent LDL from oxidizing (which makes them more damaging to arteries). The best way to balance the ratio is to eat fewer foods that contain omega-6 fatty acids and more that contain omega-3 fatty acids, such as salmon and seaweed. Some plant foods, such as flaxseeds and green leafy vegetables, contain alpha linoleic acid (ALA), an omega-3 fatty acid that converts in small amounts to EPA and DHA. However, because there is only about a 5 percent conversion of ALA to EPA and DHA, plant-based foods shouldn't be considered a reliable source. Grass-fed, free-range meat has 4 to 6 percent EPA and DHA and much lower levels of omega-6 fatty acids and saturated fats than factory-farmed meat. You can also help ensure a healthy omega balance by taking fish oil supplements.

Unsaturated Fats

Unsaturated fats are considered *good* fats because they contribute to heart and brain health and are essential to decreasing the risk of heart disease, normalizing blood clotting, balancing blood sugar, and decreasing LDL cholesterol. There are two kinds of unsaturated fats: polyunsaturated and monounsaturated. In moderation, both have a place in a healthy diet. Both are found in plant foods such as olive oil and nuts. Both help lower LDL (bad cholesterol) and raise HDL (good cholesterol).

Saturated Fats

Saturated fats can be bad *and* good. While they are commonly known as *bad* fats, the science is still unclear about the overall effect of saturated fats on heart health. This is partially because there is more than one kind of saturated fat and they aren't all equal in the health equation. Here's why:

- *Stearic acid* is a long-chain fatty acid found in meat and chocolate. Although it is a saturated fat, it has *not* been shown to cause the cardiovascular problems usually attributed to other saturated fats.
- *Lauric, capric, and caprylic acids* are medium-chain fatty acids found in coconut, which, although saturated, have shown many

health benefits. They aren't believed to have the negative effects of other saturated fats.

- *Palmitic acid* is also a saturated fat. This is what we think of as *bad* saturated fat because it has a negative impact on cholesterol and heart health. This is the fat that is created in your liver when you eat a high-sugar, high-carbohydrate diet. It also creates the cherished fat "marbling" in the meat of corn-fed cattle.
- *Myristic acid* is a saturated fat found in most animal fats, butter, and some vegetable oils. There is some evidence that this fatty acid can be detrimental to heart health and should be consumed only in small amounts.

Saturated fats have been condemned for years because of the connection between saturated fat consumption and increased cholesterol. However, current research paints a more complicated picture. Studies done on the different types of saturated fats have shown varying effects on cholesterol levels and patterns. And simply removing the saturated fats, without adding healthy fats, has not shown an improvement in heart health. Some research suggests that the healthiest strategy is to cut back on certain types of saturated fats (especially palmitic acid and myristic acid, which are found in dairy foods and meat, especially factory-farmed meat) and increase consumption of polyunsaturated fatty acids like fish oil, nuts, and seeds.

Trans Fat

Also known as trans fatty acids, trans fat really is a *bad* fat. In fact, it is the *worst* fat. It raises LDL and lowers HDL cholesterol, increases triglycerides, and increases the risk of atherosclerosis (the hardening of arteries) and heart disease, as well as of diabetes and inflammation. There is nothing positive about trans fat. It is found in many processed foods and is created when unsaturated fats are processed and chemically changed from liquid to solid form. Sources of trans fats include shortening, many margarines, many kinds of commercially prepared fried foods, and many packaged baked goods (such as doughnuts, crackers, and snack foods). Don't get too excited about the generation of trans fat–free foods hitting the shelves. Many aren't really free of trans fat. According to government regulations, trans fat doesn't have to be listed on a food label if its level is below the legal limit of 0.5 grams per serving.

It's important to realize that a single pastry is often actually several servings, even though most people will eat the whole thing in one sitting. Thus many baked goods and pastries that are in excess of 5 ounces have 2 or 3 grams of trans fat. Even small amounts of these very unhealthy fats should be avoided.

OPTIMAL VERSUS SUBOPTIMAL FATS

Optimal Fats

Avocados

Cocoa butter

Coconut

Fish: anchovies, arctic char, catfish, herring, king crab, mackerel, wild salmon, sardines, sea bass, snapper, sole, trout, and tuna

Seafood: clams, mussels, oysters, and scallops

Meats: grass-fed beef, bison, lamb, and organic poultry

Nuts

Olives

Seeds

Healthful Oils

Olive oil

Coconut oil

Avocado oil

Macadamia nut oil

Sesame oil

Walnut oil

Suboptimal or Harmful Fats

Industrial-raised animal fat and dairy

Processed meats

Trans fats

Excessive omega-6 fats

Safflower, corn, and soy oils

Canola oil

BEST OILS

Although olive oil and some other oils are nutritious when consumed in raw form, they oxidize and become harmful when heated to high temperatures. When oils reach their smoking point during cooking, they break down, lose nutritional value, and become toxic. For cooking, we usually use coconut or macadamia nut oil. These oils have a higher smoking point than olive oil, so they can get hotter without breaking down. Also note that usually you don't even need oil for cooking! Many of our recipes suggest using vegetable broth for sautéing instead of oil. In most cases, it works just as well. We recommend organic, unrefined, expeller-pressed, and cold-pressed oils. Processing strips oils of all nutritional value, leaving them as nothing more than liquid fat—and not the healthy kind. You can find unrefined oils in most health food stores. There is a detailed section on oils in *The Brain Warrior's Way Cookbook*.

Principle 6:

Eat from the Rainbow

As a Brain Warrior you want to include natural foods in your diet that reflect the full spectrum of colors and flavors, such as blueberries, pomegranates, yellow squash, and red bell peppers. This will boost the power-packed flavonoids to elevate antioxidant levels in your body and help keep your brain young.

Of course, this does not mean Skittles, jelly beans, or M&M's. It also doesn't include grape jelly, mustard (which contains food dye), or ketchup (which is usually loaded with sugar)! These highly processed, artificially colored, sugar-filled foods have no place in your pantry, in schools, or on your plate, if you are trying to use food to heal your mind and body. They do the opposite! In fact, artificial food coloring has been shown to increase symptoms of ADD. We have suggestions and delicious alternatives so that you won't miss nonnutritious foods.

THE REWARD IS IN THE RAINBOW

It's abundantly clear that colorful plant foods have tremendous health benefits. They provide an enormous array of plant nutrients, enzymes, vitamins, and minerals necessary for good health. These foods also support optimal health at the cellular level. Compounds in plant foods can help repair defects in DNA. This is important because defective DNA can lead to cancer, chronic diseases, and aging-related health conditions. For example sulforaphanes found in broccoli and other cruciferous vegetables, such as cauliflower, and various herbs and spices, such as curcumin, offer natural, powerful support in the process of DNA repair. Plant foods also help prevent cancer and reduce inflammation that contributes to Alzheimer's disease, heart disease, arthritis, gastrointestinal disorders, high blood pressure, and many other diseases.

The vast array of nutrients in fruits and vegetables boosts the health of just about every system in your body. They are rich in antioxidants, which help fight free radicals and decrease the damage they may cause. Nutrients found in plant foods—such as zinc, selenium, iron, copper, folic acid as well as vitamins A, C, E, and B_6—support a strong, disease-fighting immune system and aid in detoxification. Other chemicals found in colorful plants have been shown to be cardioprotective (lower blood pressure and prevent LDL oxidation), chemoprotective (fight many types of cancer), and neuroprotective (sequester debris in the brain associated with Alzheimer's disease).

ANTIOXIDANT-RICH FOODS
(OXYGEN RADICAL ABSORBANCE
CAPACITY, PER 100 GRAMS OF WEIGHT)

Cloves 290,000	Cocoa powder 55,000
Oregano 175,000	Raspberries 19,000
Rosemary 165,000	Walnuts 13,000
Thyme 157,000	Blueberries 9,600
Cinnamon 131,000	Artichokes 9,400
Turmeric 125,000	Cranberries 9,000
Sage 120,000	Kidney beans 8,600
Acai fruit 102,000	Blackberries 5,900
Parsley 73,000	Pomegranates 4,400

In a 2015 study, the plant medicine apigenin, found in parsley, thyme, chamomile, and red bell peppers, was found to strengthen connections between brain cells.[67] Many people think that blueberries are a classic example of an antioxidant-promoting, brain healthy fruit, but when you look at the oxygen radical absorbance capacity (ORAC) values in the table on page 129, it is clear that cloves, oregano, rosemary, thyme, cinnamon, turmeric, and sage lead the way for antioxidant power.

Principle 7:

Cook with Brain Healthy Herbs and Spices

SPICES: TO LIVE AND DIE FOR

When you think of herbs and spices, you probably think of the strange little bottles in the corner of your kitchen collecting dust. Or maybe spices conjure exotic images of flavorful food from faraway lands. Spices probably don't make you think of war.

From the beginning of time, humans started their search for ways to preserve food, heal wounds, and extend life. This quest yielded quick and powerful results from tribes around the globe, in the form of herbs and spices. In fact, herbs and spices were so effectively used as medicine, food preservation, building strength, and even as aphrodisiacs that people went on life-threatening explorations in search of more and different spices. Trade routes were planned around spices, many of which were worth more than jewels and silk. Many wars throughout history have even been fought over spices. One of the most famous of these wars was the Spice Wars of the 1500s, fought over nutmeg, which was thought to be a cure for the plague. The Portuguese first fought the Dutch, who later fought the English for this pungent medicinal seasoning. This wasn't the first war, and it wouldn't be the last in the quest to obtain spices believed to heal all that was ailing people around the world.

Herbs and spices were believed to be so powerful and to have so many uses that they were sometimes used as ransom payments by armies during wartime. They could also buy a slave's freedom. Documentation from the fourteenth century showed that in Germany 1 pound of nutmeg could be traded for seven fat oxen.

Hippocrates listed over 500 medicinal uses for herbs and spices, including ways to prevent illness and increase longevity. It's no wonder people have been willing to fight for these precious miracle plant substances. Unlike pharmaceutical drugs, which often come with an alarming range of warnings about possible side effects, herbs and spices generally have minimal consequences, often limited to rare allergic reactions. They're also comparatively inexpensive and don't require the approval of a health insurer.

About 80 percent of the developing world still relies on natural and herbal remedies as their primary source of medicines. It is likely not a coincidence that even though the United States spends more money on health care than any other country on earth, Americans rank *twenty-eighth* in overall health and *twenty-fourth* in life expectancy!

Although they are chemically processed, most of today's medications are derived from plant sources. For example, opium and many other pain medications are derived from poppy seeds, quinine comes from cinchona bark, and the cancer drug vincristine comes from periwinkle. Aspirin (salicylic acid), our primary pain reliever for more than 150 years, is derived from willow bark, meadowsweet, and ulmaria.

Herbs and spices are one of the few food categories that provide *both* nutrition and flavor. This is what we call win–win—food that serves your health and excites your taste buds—and if you're a Brain Warrior, you like to *win*! Herbs and spices contain so many health-promoting substances that it almost makes sense to store them in the medicine cabinet rather than in the spice cabinet! The seasonings we use in cooking, and often take for granted, are derived from some of the same plants for which our ancestors risked their lives to obtain pain relief, vitality, and healing. Let's say you take them out, dust them off and start improving your health and the taste of your food. The only fight you will have to engage in is the line at the grocery store. There is a detailed section about spices in *The Brain Warrior's Way Cookbook* with delicious ways to serve them up.

WHAT'S BEHIND THE HEALING POWER OF HERBS AND SPICES?

- **Antioxidants** give herbs and spices the ability to bind to free radicals and to aid in the repair of DNA and the prevention of cancer.
- **Phytoalexins** are plant compounds that are toxic in high doses, but cancer preventive in low doses. Think of these like mini chemo agents.

(CONTINUED)

- **Polyphenols** are compounds that contribute to the color, flavor, bitterness, and odor of plant foods. They have powerful antioxidant and anti-inflammatory properties.
- **Carotenoids** are a source of antioxidants that are high in vitamin A. These powerful cancer fighters are also hailed for their immune-boosting abilities.
- **Fiber** such as glucans, glycans, and lignans found in herbs and other plant foods helps regulate hormones and boost immunity.
- **Organominerals** have antioxidant, anti-inflammatory, and antimicrobial properties.
- **Alkaloids** are nitrogen-containing compounds. Some, like caffeine, are psychoactive, while others are antimicrobial and anti-inflammatory by nature.

Here are a handful of our favorite herbs and spices, with a few of their benefits. For a complete list, see *The Brain Warrior's Way Cookbook*.

- Turmeric, found in curry, contains a chemical that has been shown to decrease the plaques in the brain thought to be responsible for Alzheimer's disease.
- In multiple studies, a saffron extract was found to be as effective as antidepressant medication in treating people with major depression.
- Scientific evidence shows rosemary, thyme, and sage help boost memory.
- Cinnamon has been shown to help improve attention and blood sugar regulation. It is high in antioxidants and is a natural aphrodisiac.
- Garlic and oregano boost blood flow to the brain.
- The hot, spicy taste of ginger, cayenne, and black pepper comes from gingerols, capsaicin, and piperine—compounds that boost metabolism and have an aphrodisiac effect.

Principle 8:

Make Sure Your Food Is as Clean as Possible

The food sitting in your refrigerator at this very moment will have a monumental impact on your health, either for better or for worse. You can positively change the action of your brain, immune system, hormones, genes, and blood sugar with clean, nutrient-dense food. In many cases, food can be as effective as, or even much more effective than, pharmaceutical medications. Relying on multiple medicines to heal conditions that are being caused by excessive consumption of inflammation-inducing foods is like putting a Band-Aid over a gunshot wound. Eventually it's going to give out!

Whenever possible, eat organically grown or raised foods, as pesticides used in commercial farming can accumulate in your brain and body, even though the levels in each food may be low. Also, choose to eat hormone-free, antibiotic-free meat from animals that are free range and grass fed whenever you can. As the Apache warriors would say, you are not only what you eat—you are also what the animals you eat ate. In addition and as much as possible, eliminate food additives, preservatives, and artificial dyes and sweeteners. To do so, you must start reading food labels. If you do not know what is in a food item or product, don't eat it. Would you ever spend money on something if you did not know the cost? Of course not. Now is the time to become thoughtful and serious about the food you put in your body.

The standard American diet is filled with chemical-laden, antibiotic- and hormone-filled, proinflammatory foods. Fast food, sugar, simple carbohydrates, dairy products, trans fats, some animal-derived saturated fats, and excess omega-6 fatty acids as well as foods that are processed, engineered, or refined promote chronic inflammation in your body and brain. When you eat food that contains chemicals that are unnatural to you, your body sees it as an "injury." Inflammation is how your body tries to heal itself. In other words, you're forcing your body into a chronic state of emergency trying to recover from harm.

Fortunately, you can fight back by choosing clean food; foods that reduce inflammation, such as fresh organic vegetables and fruits (when possible), wild fish that are rich in omega-3s, nuts, seeds, and certain herbs and spices. In fact, your brain and body are so hungry for nutrient-dense healing foods that most people notice remarkable changes within a matter of weeks. So even if you've been living an unhealthy lifestyle, it's not too late to change!

We understand that most people cannot afford to eat everything organic and sustainably raised. The Environmental Working Group produces a list every year of the foods that are imperative to eat organic, and those which are not as important to be organic. You can stay updated at ewg.org. Here is the current list.

FOODS WITH THE HIGHEST LEVELS OF PESTICIDE RESIDUES (BUY ORGANIC OR DON'T EAT THEM)

1. Celery
2. Peaches
3. Apples
4. Blueberries
5. Cucumbers
6. Sweet bell peppers
7. Cherries
8. Collard greens/kale
9. Grapes
10. Green beans
11. Strawberries
12. Nectarines
13. Spinach
14. Potatoes

FOODS WITH THE LOWEST LEVELS OF PESTICIDE RESIDUES

1. Onions
2. Pineapples
3. Sweet peas (frozen)
4. Cabbage
5. Mushrooms
6. Eggplant
7. Avocado
8. Mango
9. Kiwi
10. Broccoli
11. Watermelon
12. Cantaloupe
13. Asparagus
14. Bananas
15. Papaya
16. Grapefruit

Fish is a great source of healthy protein and fat as mentioned earlier, but it's important to consider the toxicity in some fish. Here are a couple of general rules to guide you in choosing more healthful fish:

1. The larger the fish, the more mercury it may contain, so go for the smaller varieties.

2. From the safe fish choices, eat a fairly wide variety of fish, preferably those highest in omega-3s, like wild Alaskan salmon, sardines, anchovies, hake, and haddock.

You can also learn more at seafoodwatch.org.

Believe it or not, the greatest danger from antibiotics does not come from those prescribed by your doctor but rather from the foods you eat. The prevalence of antibiotics found in conventionally raised meats and vegetables has the potential to throw off the balance of good to bad gut bacteria. It is estimated that 70 percent of the total antibiotic use in the United States is for livestock. Again, try to focus on eating foods that are antibiotic-free, hormone-free, grass-fed, and free-range.

Principle 9:

Eliminate Any Potential Allergens or Internal Attackers

Did you know that for some people gluten can literally mess with their mind? There are scientific reports of people having psychotic episodes or feeling anxious or depressed when they've ingested gluten.[68] When these people eliminate wheat and other gluten sources (such as barley, rye, spelt, imitation meats, and soy sauce) from their diets, their stomachs and their brains function better.

We have many, many stories of patients who lose weight and completely eliminate brain fog, irritability, eczema, and irritable bowel symptoms when they get gluten out of their diet. One of our patients would become violent whenever he ate MSG. When we scanned him on MSG, his brain changed into a pattern more consistent with our aggressive patients. This is important: MSG doesn't have to be labeled unless it is a single food additive. It can be disguised by being added in with other ingredients and not disclosed. It is commonly hidden in bouillon, soy protein isolate, vegetable protein isolate, and whey protein isolate.

Children with ADHD and on the autism spectrum often feel and behave better when we put them on diets that get rid of wheat (and all food containing gluten), dairy, corn, soy, processed foods, all forms of sugar and sugar alternatives, food dyes, and additives.

You can take blood tests to learn more about your sensitivities to food, but we have found the "poor man's test" (simply eliminating certain foods and slowly adding them back in) is very effective. In Part 7, we give you detailed instructions for an elimination diet. It is how we start Brain Warrior Basic Training and the 14-Day Brain Boost.

If you really want to get and stay healthy, it is critical you start choosing foods that serve your health and lose the ones that steal from it. Using the ten Brain Warrior Nutrition Principles, we will show you the foods to choose and the ones to lose to optimize your brain and body for the rest of your life.

Principle 10:

Eat Healthfully During the Day, but Fast 12 Hours at Night

It is critical to start the day with breakfast to stabilize your blood sugar and jump-start your metabolism. In the morning, make sure to include some healthy fat in your meal to prevent cravings later in the day and also help you better absorb your vitamins.

Throughout the day, it is critical to eat healthy food and never allow your blood sugar to go too low. Otherwise, your cravings can hijack your decision-making abilities, and you're more likely to make bad choices. The following is a list of hypoglycemic (low blood sugar) symptoms:

- Feeling sleepy/drugged
- Mental confusion
- Inability to concentrate
- Impaired memory
- Dizzy, light-headed
- Nervousness
- Depression
- Anger, irritability
- Anxiety/panic attacks
- Palpitations
- Shaky hands
- Butterflies in the stomach
- Flushing/sweating

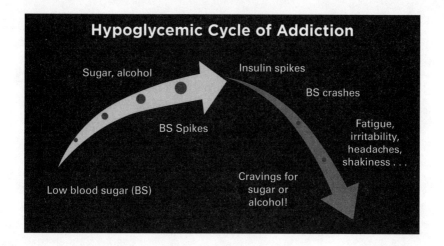

Hypoglycemic Cycle of Addiction

Sugar, alcohol

Insulin spikes

BS crashes

BS Spikes

Fatigue, irritability, headaches, shakiness . . .

Cravings for sugar or alcohol!

Low blood sugar (BS)

- Frontal headache
- Insomnia
- Abdominal pain/diarrhea

If you have two or three of these symptoms, make sure to have three to five small meals throughout the day. One of our patients kept getting into fights at work and ended up getting arrested. His glucose tolerance test showed a remarkable drop in blood sugar 2 hours after he had consumed a sugar load. When we balanced his diet with frequent healthy meals, his behavior and temper were much better.

It is also important to fast for at least 12 hours each night, between the last food in the evening and the first in the morning. Begin the fasting at least 3 hours before bedtime. Some occasional daytime fasts may also be helpful, such as fasting for a day (or most of a day) every few months. This will help your body in many ways, especially for memory. Memory loss may be observed in people producing too much beta amyloid plaque, which readily turns toxic in the brain. A critical mechanism for clearing these plaques is via something called autophagy, which you can think of like tiny Pac-Men cleaning up the trash. Nightly fasts (and the occasional daytime fast) can nudge certain mechanisms in your brain to induce autophagy and clean up beta amyloid and other troublemaking proteins.

FOODS TO CHOOSE

BRAIN HEALTHY FOODS TO BOOST YOUR MENTAL, EMOTIONAL AND COGNITIVE ABILITIES

To help you get started on the right path, here is our list of the 100 best brain healthy superfoods that fit all ten of the Brain Warrior Nutrition Principles. Often, when people find out what they shouldn't eat, they'll say, "But there isn't anything left to eat. I'll starve." We can guarantee you won't starve. In fact, there are hundreds of healthy and delicious foods you can eat. Here are a hundred of our favorite brain healthy ones to choose.

Beverages

1. Water
2. Sparkling water, plain or with a splash of flavored stevia
3. Green tea
4. Coconut water

Nuts and Seeds

5. Almonds, raw
6. Brazil nuts
7. Macadamia nuts
8. Cacao, raw
9. Cashews
10. Chia seeds
11. Coconut
12. Flaxseeds
13. Hemp seeds
14. Pistachios
15. Pumpkin seeds
16. Quinoa
17. Sesame seeds
18. Walnuts

Legumes (Small Amounts—Eat Them like a Condiment)

19. Lentils
20. Chickpeas
21. Sugar snap peas or snow peas

Fruits

22. Acai berries
23. Apples

24. Avocados
25. Blackberries
26. Black currants
27. Blueberries
28. Cherries
29. Cranberries
30. Golden berries
31. Goji berries
32. Grapefruits
33. Kiwis
34. Lemons
35. Limes
36. Peaches
37. Plums
38. Pomegranates
39. Raspberries
40. Strawberries

Vegetables

41. Artichokes
42. Asparagus
43. Bell peppers
44. Beets
45. Bok choy
46. Broccoli
47. Brussels sprouts
48. Butternut squash
49. Cabbage
50. Cauliflower
51. Celery
52. Chlorella
53. Collard greens
54. Fermented vegetables, such as fresh sauerkraut and kimchi (pickled cabbage, garlic, ginger and red peppers)
55. Kale
56. Leeks
57. Onions
58. Seaweed
59. Spinach
60. Spirulina
61. Sweet potatoes

Oils

62. Avocado oil
63. Coconut oil
64. Macadamia nut oil
65. Olive oil

Meats (When Possible Try to Get Grass-Fed, Hormone-Free, Antibiotic-Free, Free-Range, Harvested Humanely)

66. Chicken
67. Eggs
68. Turkey
69. Bison
70. Beef
71. Pork
72. Lamb

Seafood

73. Anchovies
74. Black cod
75. Hake
76. Haddock
77. Oysters
78. Halibut
79. Mackerel (avoid King Mackerel, high in mercury)
80. Rainbow trout
81. Salmon, Wild Alaskan
82. Sardines
83. Dungeness crab

Spices

84. Basil (sweet, dried)
85. Cinnamon
86. Cloves
87. Garlic
88. Oregano
89. Rosemary
90. Saffron
91. Sage
92. Thyme
93. Turmeric
94. Nutmeg

Sweeteners (Avoid Sugar in All Forms, Including Agave and Fruit Juices, and the Artificial Sweeteners Aspartame, Sucralose, and Saccharin)

95. Stevia
96. Erythritol
97. Xylitol
98. Honey, raw, wild (small amounts only)

Special Category

99. Shirataki noodles
100. Maca root

FOODS THAT MAKE YOU SMARTER AND HAPPIER

Eating the Brain Warrior's Way will give you more than a warrior's body. It will literally change the way you think and just may improve all aspects of your life. The quality of your diet *directly impacts* the quality of your life. The lens through which you see the world is heavily influenced and tinted by everything you put in your mouth. A fast-food, processed diet actually changes the chemistry and function of your brain. If you feel depressed, foggy, unmotivated, and disempowered, it may not all be psychological. Food has influence over six major neurotransmitters in the brain.

Serotonin, the "don't worry, be happy" neurotransmitter, is responsible for mood stability, sleep regulation, appetite control, and social engagement. Serotonin levels go down (sometimes dramatically) at certain times in a woman's menstrual cycle, making her irritable and even depressed. Being low in serotonin is a common cause of depression and anxiety. If you know someone who gets stuck on negative thoughts and can't let go, it could be a sign of low serotonin.

People who are naturally low in serotonin often intuitively crave carbohydrate-rich foods such as pasta, bread, and sugar-filled chocolate because carbohydrates raise serotonin levels and *temporarily* increase feelings of well-being. If you're in need of some serotonin-boosting carbs, however, you don't have to reach for refined carbohydrates that trigger inflammation, blood sugar spikes, and high insulin. Complex carbs from plant foods like sweet potatoes and apples, or a square of sugar-free dark chocolate can help. The following supplements also help: 5-HTP, inositol, and saffron.

HAPPINESS: TWELVE SMART CARBS TO BOOST SEROTONIN

1. Sweet potatoes
2. Hummus
3. Apples
4. Pears
5. Peaches
6. Blueberries
7. Bananas
8. Oranges or tangerines
9. Grapes
10. Figs
11. Mangoes
12. Pineapples

Did you know that nearly 90 percent of the serotonin in your body is made in your gut? So if you are suffering from digestive issues and intestinal permeability, you will likely have other issues related to serotonin imbalance. Women take note: A study from McGill University in Canada found that women have a 52 percent lower production rate of serotonin than men do, which could explain why women report twice as much depression as men *and why they crave simple carbohydrates and chocolate!* And unfortunately, birth control pills often lead to further reduction in serotonin. It's no wonder that women are twice as likely to suffer from depression. Exercise and smart carbohydrates can make a big difference in your mood, mind, and body.

WHY RESTAURANTS GIVE YOU FREE BREAD AND PUSH ALCOHOL BEFORE MEALS

Why do restaurants serve free baskets of bread before each meal? Why not cheese? Why not almonds or chunks of beef or chicken? The reason is that bread makes you hungrier and encourages you to eat more. Bread quickly spikes your blood sugar, which boosts the hormone insulin. Insulin then drives the amino acid tryptophan, which is the precursor for serotonin, into the brain, making people feel happier and more relaxed. Unfortunately, it also drops the function of your prefrontal cortex (your brain's supervisor), making you more impulsive. In addition, servers push alcohol at the beginning of a meal, which also lowers the judgment centers in the brain. If you eat bread and drink alcohol before a meal, you are much more likely to order dessert, even though when you entered the restaurant you told yourself you wouldn't.

Dopamine is the neurotransmitter associated with motivation, emotional significance, relevance, focus, and the ability to experience pleasure. Dopamine-dominant people are usually focused go-getters and a little intense; a lack of dopamine is associated with ADD, lack of focus, and lower motivation.

Protein-rich foods such as seafood, poultry, and lean meat help boost dopamine. This is why high-protein diets that eliminate refined carbohydrates are ideal for people with ADD. However, when people with low serotonin go on a high-protein, low-carb diet, they can quickly find themselves unable to sleep and can be overfocused on certain thoughts—especially stressful ones that they can't let go of. The following supplements are good for people who are low in dopamine: green tea, ashwagandha, rhodiola, ginseng, and L-tyrosine.

BEST FOODS TO BOOST DOPAMINE, ENERGY, AND FOCUS

1. Beans—lima beans and lentils
2. Meat—fish, lamb, chicken, turkey and beef
3. Eggs
4. Nuts
5. Seeds—pumpkin and sesame
6. High-protein veggies—broccoli and spinach
7. Protein powders

Acetylcholine is a critical neurotransmitter for learning, memory, and association. Lack of acetylcholine can lead to declining cognitive function and difficulty learning new information. To stay sharp, eat foods that optimize acetylcholine, including eggs, liver, lecithin, salmon, and shrimp. Helpful supplements include choline, phosphatidylcholine, and lecithin.

GABA is an inhibitory neurotransmitter. It is calming, stabilizing, and grounding. It has the opposite effect of dopamine. Think of dopamine like the "gas" and GABA like the "brake." Decreased GABA is associated with anxiety, irritability, and some cyclic mood issues, like bipolar disorder. Foods that are rich in GABA include broccoli, nuts, and lentils. Supplements include GABA, Relora, and L-theanine.

Glutamate and **aspartate** are excitatory neurotransmitters associated with memory, learning, and pain perception. However, consumed in excess they are potent neurotoxins. The standard American diet has an overabundance of foods that contain the amino acids that stimulate these neurotransmitters, including the artificial sweetener aspartame, processed lunch meat, sausage, soy, wheat, peanuts, monosodium glutamate (MSG), and some preservatives. Having too much of these neurotransmitters damages neurons, causes cell death, and is associated with stroke and diseases, such as amyotrophic lateral sclerosis (ALS), autism spectrum disorders, intellectual disability, and Alzheimer's disease. It's no wonder that we've seen a sharp increase in the incidence of neurodegenerative disease and other brain-related problems, given the declining standard of nutrition in our country.

Understanding your brain and simple biochemistry will help you thrive, especially knowing which foods to choose.

BRAIN WARRIORS ARE VALUE DRIVEN

"I can't afford to be healthy," is a refrain we hear almost every day. We'll grant you that buying 1,000 calories of Cocoa Puffs is cheaper than buying 1,000 calories of fresh vegetables or pasture-raised meat. And if you're trying to support yourself and your family on limited funds, it can be difficult to choose a fresh avocado at $1.29 instead of the gooey, green, prepackaged and preserved "avocado sauce" that probably doesn't contain an ounce of avocado.

There's no doubt about it—we live in a broken food culture where the weapons of mass destruction pervade. Government subsidies support the production of cheap, low-quality foods that make us sick, fat, and depressed. The first thing you see as you walk into the store are miles of aisles filled with chemically manufactured foods that are purposely designed to attract your attention and condition your taste buds to eat even more sugar, bad fat, and salt in larger and larger quantities. It's not always easy to choose salad greens and fish if you aren't a warrior on a mission.

You have to be armed and ready with a strategy for eating healthy on a budget. Yes, it may mean changing your habits and priorities a bit, but we assure you the results will be worth it.

Here are 30 tips to make the BWW sustenance plan easy and inexpensive.

1. When you start eating healthy Brain Warrior foods you will save a great deal of money by not eating the unhealthy ones. You will save on the dozens of charges for the expensive sugar-filled coffee drinks, muffins, pastries, and impulsive bad-food purchases.
2. Buy a water filter to have an unlimited supply of clean water. You can buy faucet filters for around $20 or under-the-counter reverse-osmosis filters for less than $200.
3. Don't buy drinks. This can be a huge savings. Drink water or make spa water with a few orange, tangerine, or cucumber slices in a water jug (yes, as if you were in an expensive hotel in Hawaii).
4. Shop online, compare prices. Several Internet retailers have apps where you can scan labels in a store and see if you can get the item cheaper online. Many online re-

tailers also have free shipping, so you are also saving on gas and time (time is money).

5. Plan your meals and shopping trips. Be a mindful shopper and make a list before you go to the store, which will help limit impulsive buying.

6. Shop *after* you have eaten. Hungry shoppers have higher grocery bills, because they have lower blood sugar and lower blood flow to their frontal lobes.

7. Buy whole foods, the ones that *grow* on a plant, rather than those *made* in a plant and undoctored seafood, poultry, and meat. This way you have complete control over the ingredients, and they are often less expensive. Avoid anything that comes from a box as much as you possibly can. Examples of whole foods are
   - Proteins: healthful meats, fish, and eggs
   - Carbs: veggies, fruits and sweet potatoes
   - Fats: olive oil, seeds, nuts and avocados.

8. Prepare in bulk and use throughout the week. Bulk foods are often cheaper, but make sure not to waste them. For example, healthful turkey can make a great meal and can be reused in salads, soups, and wraps.

9. Shop for fruits and vegetables that are in season because they are fresher and more affordable. Plus you can freeze anything extra to save money year round. These foods are loaded with antioxidants and fiber. Go with the low-glycemic, high-fiber ones, especially organic berries, kale, cabbage, spinach, cauliflower, and broccoli.

10. Buy frozen fruits and vegetables. You are more likely to use them all, and there is less chance of having spoiled produce that must be thrown away. The freezing process does remove some of the vitamin content, but frozen vegetables are still an inexpensive way to get brain-boosting, antiaging, disease-fighting nutrients.

11. Become freezer happy. If you have something about to go bad, figure out a way to freeze it so you have minimal waste.

(CONTINUED)

12. Pump up protein with affordable eggs; this is one of our favorite ways to obtain high-quality calories that pack a protein power punch.

13. Buy whole chickens rather than parts of chickens. It is more cost effective and can save you up to 75 percent.

14. Spice up your foods. Spices have brain benefits as discussed earlier and you only have to buy them infrequently, which makes them affordable. You can also purchase spices in bulk and create your own blends, making them much cheaper.

15. Go to your local farmers' markets, where you can get locally grown food that is often organic and high-quality at a reasonable price, because there is no middle man. Websites like Local Harvest and Eat Well Guide can help you find a Community Supported Agriculture (CSA) farmer or farmers' market in your area. Websites like Eat Wild have resources for finding a local supplier of grass-fed beef or other healthful meats and the like.

16. Buy generic brands when possible. They are usually made by the brand name companies but sell for less.

17. Plan for leftovers. When making meals, purposely make enough extra food for lunch the next day.

18. When choosing organic, spend money on the more contaminated (that is, pesticide laden) foods and less on nonorganic from the least contaminated list.

19. Buy raw nuts in bulk and divide them up into smaller portions. Freezing nuts is also a good strategy; they are cheaper in bulk and stay freshest in the freezer.

20. Join together with friends to buy a whole or half a cow or pig from a nearby farmer who doesn't use antibiotics or hormones on the animals. There's an initial investment for the deep freezer and the bulk meat, but it pays off in the end.

21. Ground turkey and larger bags of hormone-free chicken thighs and legs are often inexpensive, yet nutritious.

22. Organic frozen tilapia (bought in bulk) is a fabulous fish that cooks in no time and is usually very affordable. Just sprinkle it with a little of your favorite seasoning on one side and sauté it in a small amount of coconut oil.

Squeeze a slice of citrus on top, and dinner is served. This is also great for fish tacos.

23. Use some high-fiber, low-cost beans. Also high in protein, beans should be a staple in any household that is struggling financially. To be extra economical, choose uncooked black beans, red beans, garbanzo beans, white beans, or any other variety, rather than canned beans.

24. Check newspapers and online sites for specials and, if the foods meet the ten principles, include them on your shopping list.

25. When the waiter asks you if you want alcohol before a meal, say no. Order seltzer and put a few drops of flavored stevia in it (SweetLeaf is our favorite brand). It's generally cost-free as well as calorie-free!

26. Skip the appetizers in restaurants. They just add unneeded calories.

27. Split meals in restaurants. The portions are usually too big anyway.

28. Join a local food co-op.

29. Stop going out to eat. Making your own meals increases your nutrition and is much more cost effective.

30. Grow your own food. It will be more nutritious and give you more purpose in your life.

THIRTEEN SUPER BRAIN FOODS FOR LESS THAN $1 PER SERVING

1. Lentils
2. Kale, spinach
3. Broccoli
4. Red bell peppers
5. Almonds
6. Tea
7. Oranges
8. Tuna
9. Sweet potatoes
10. Apples
11. Eggs
12. Black beans
13. Cabbage

FOODS TO LOSE

In our experience, some foods are not worth the downsides that come along with them, and some are clearly weapons of mass destruction.

There are foods we feel you should limit or avoid altogether, including sugar, artificial sweeteners, gluten, soy, corn, and dairy. These foods are prevalent in most diets and yet they cause myriad symptoms that can affect your overall brain function and health.

SUGAR: SWEET DEATH

Sugar is not your friend. One study from the University of California, San Francisco (UCSF) found that sugary soda had the same negative impact on your cells as cigarettes and was associated with accelerated aging.[69] Robert Lustig, a pediatric endocrinologist from UCSF, flatly states that sugar is addictive and it is the *primary* cause of obesity, hypertension, heart disease, cholesterol problems, and diabetes—all of which cause brain damage.[70] He says that fructose is particularly troublesome, as it is processed in the liver like alcohol. If you watch Lustig's 90-minute YouTube video, *Sugar: The Bitter Truth*, you will be much less likely to ever drink fruit juice again.[71]

Refined sugar is 99.4 to 99.7 percent pure calories, with no vitamins, minerals, fats, or proteins—just carbohydrates that spike blood sugar, followed by an insulin response and a subsequent sugar crash, leading us to the desire for more. Eating sugary foods makes people hungry and tired, and causes them to gain weight. Refined sugar is void of minerals needed for enzymes, can cause mineral deficiencies, interferes with the actions of calcium and magnesium, increases inflammation, increases erratic brain cell firing, and has been implicated in aggression. Sugar consumption has been associated with depression, ADHD and hyperactivity, increased triglycerides, lower HDL, and higher LDL cholesterol; it also feeds cancer cells. Brain imaging studies showed sugar causes increased slow brain waves, and a study at UCLA showed that sugar alters learning and memory.[72] On average Americans eat about 140 pounds of sugar a year.

When Daniel turned fifty, three different people bought him cakes. His response was "Don't you want me to be sixty?" One has to wonder why we celebrate with something that clearly hurts us. Sugar (ice cream, candy, or cakes) is used to celebrate birthdays, weddings, anniversaries, graduations, promotions, holidays, and the end of a meal. When we are young, we are taught that sweets are for soothing hurts, celebrating successes, and drowning our sorrows. There always seems to be a reason to hurt ourselves.

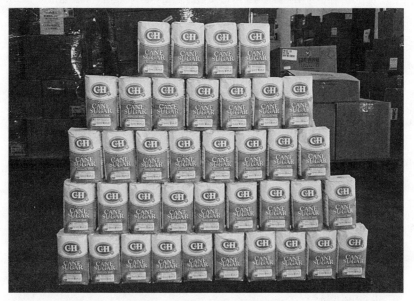

Advertisers are masterful at convincing people that if something is natural it must be good. Nightshade berries and death cap mushrooms are natural—and they will kill you. The fact that sugar is often disguised behind the labels of "organic," "cane," "raw," or "unprocessed" doesn't change the insulin response in your body when you eat it. Whether it comes from a beehive, a maple tree, or any other natural source, sugar is sugar. When you eat sugar, your blood sugar spikes, insulin is released, then blood sugar drops, and you crave it again and again. When your blood sugar drops, your body sees it as a state of emergency, causing you to crave food as a way to fix the situation. Sugar is the fastest way to do that. That is why when you eat sugar and simple carbs, you crave them, like a drug addict craves his drug.

All forms of sugar spike insulin regardless of the source, but some are less toxic to the liver than others. Raw honey and unprocessed forms of sugar lack the chemical processing and bleaching process. Raw, unfiltered honey contains trace amounts of minerals and vitamins, and has shown some promise in aiding in the treatment of environmental allergies (*in small amounts*). Filtering and pasteurizing honey kills the bacteria, but it also kills any nutritional or antibacterial benefits you would receive. *Never give honey (especially raw and unfiltered) to a child under the age of one year. The bacteria could cause botulism.*

Pure maple syrup also has trace minerals and significant amounts of zinc and manganese, so it is slightly preferable to table sugar. But use caution when purchasing maple syrup. Because it is expensive to manufacture, many companies have figured out cheap ways to capitalize on this tasty syrup. Most pancake syrups have no maple in them at all (hence the name "pancake syrup")—they are primarily made of high-fructose corn syrup and artificial flavoring. They are truly atrocious for your health. Choose grade B maple syrup for higher trace minerals and use it in small amounts.

Avoid agave, because of its high fructose content (it varies depending on its source, but it is generally 80 to 90 percent fructose—yikes!). Agave has been hyped as the best sweetener for people with diabetes. Fructose doesn't cause the same insulin spike reaction as sucrose, so it is often referred to as a low-glycemic sweetener. That is true, but it is toxic to the liver and can ultimately lead to metabolic syndrome, fatty liver, and insulin resistance. Agave should be avoided or used in very small amounts.

YOUR DIET EITHER HELPS HEALING FROM BRAIN INJURIES OR HURTS IT

Research from UCLA in 2015 showed that high-sugar diets sabotaged the brain's ability to heal from traumatic brain injuries (TBIs).[73] This is important news for TBI sufferers, veterans, athletes, and patients diagnosed with diseases like Parkinson's and those recovering from a stroke. Your diet is a vital part of the recovery process and can either encourage healing or impair it. According to the CDC, nearly 2 million people suffer a TBI every year. The UCLA study looked at rats trained to escape a maze over a period of five days. They were randomly assigned to two groups—one fed regular water, the other fed water laced with fructose for six weeks, simulating a human diet high in sugar. One week later the rats were given a TBI while under anesthesia. After six weeks, the researchers tested the rats' ability to remember the maze. The rats fed the regular water completed the maze with no problem, while those fed sugar water took 30 percent longer to find their way out.

According to Fernando Gomez-Pinilla, at UCLA's David Geffen School of Medicine and Brain Injury Research Center, "The sweetener interfered with the ability of neurons to communicate with each other, rewire connections after injury, record memories and produce enough energy to fuel basic functions. That's a huge obstacle for anyone to overcome—but especially for a TBI patient, who is often struggling to relearn daily routines and how to care for himself or herself. . . . Our findings suggest that fructose disrupts plasticity—the creation of fresh pathways between brain cells that occurs when we learn or experience something new."

KNOW THE TOP FOURTEEN NAMES FOR SUGAR

1. Sugar
2. Molasses
3. Caramel color
4. Barley malt
5. Corn syrup
6. Corn syrup solids
7. High-fructose corn syrup
8. Honey
9. Sorbitol
10. Fructose
11. Cane juice crystals
12. Maltose
13. Fruit juice concentrate
14. Maltodextrin

HIDDEN SUGARS

Sugar is hidden in many places. You have to read the labels if you are going to protect yourself. Sugar is often found in:

- Alcoholic beverages
- Ketchup—accounting for almost half of the calories in it
- Most luncheon meats
- Breading on many products
- Most store-bought breads
- Many salad dressings
- Hamburgers—often added to prevent shrinkage
- Fast-food grilled chicken

TOP TWENTY CARBOHYDRATES IN THE HARVARD NURSES' HEALTH STUDY

Take a look at the top twenty carbohydrates consumed in the United States. Do you see any healthful ones?

1.	Potatoes	11.	Cookies, pastries
2.	White bread	12.	Other fruit juices
3.	Breakfast cereal	13.	Coca-Cola
4.	Dark bread	14.	Apples
5.	Orange juice	15.	Skim milk
6.	Bananas	16.	Pancakes
7.	White rice	17.	Table sugar
8.	Pizza	18.	Jam
9.	Pasta	19.	French fries
10.	Muffins	20.	Candy

SWEET NOTHINGS: WHAT ABOUT ARTIFICIAL SWEETENERS?

Philosophically, replacing sugar with artificial sweeteners sounds logical. For decades it's been the general belief that artificial sweeteners have fewer calories, so they should be eaten with abandon. Except not when it comes to your health. We commend you for making an effort to eat less sugar, but like so many things that seem too good to be true, artificial sweeteners haven't turned out to be a miracle. They don't lead to significant reductions in calorie intake or dramatically lower blood sugar levels. *But they do fill your body with chemicals that can negatively affect your brain.* The big promises made about artificial sweeteners have turned out to be sweet little lies.

Artificial sweeteners have been shown to *elevate* insulin levels because they send a signal to the brain that "something sweet is coming." So although they don't elevate blood sugar, they can still raise blood insulin levels. Consuming artificial sweeteners on a regular basis can contribute to chronically high insulin, which increases your risk for Alzheimer's disease and raises the risk of heart disease, diabetes, metabolic syndrome, and other health problems. In addition, insulin is a fat-storing hormone, meaning that the presence of insulin signals your body to hold fat.

Artificial sweeteners also don't lead to weight loss. In fact, they may lower metabolism, leading to weight *gain*. In research studies, rats fed artificially sweetened foods have been found to have slower metabolisms and greater weight gain than those given sugar-sweetened foods—despite the fact that the rats who ate sugary foods consumed more calories than those who ate artificially sweetened foods. A contributing factor for weight gain in humans is that when people eat "sugar-free" foods, they believe they can consume larger quantities—and they usually do!

Most artificial sweeteners are created by a chemical process that requires the use of strong chemicals, some of which are known to harm the body, and many which have unknown long-term effects.

Here are some of the most common artificial sweeteners.

Aspartame (brand names NutraSweet and Equal) is the world's bestselling artificial sweetener found in a great many foods, including soft drinks, chewing gums, and sugar-free candies. It has been responsible for a high number of complaints to the U.S. Food and Drug Administration (FDA),[74] including headaches, memory loss, depression, gastrointestinal distress, chronic pain, and violent rages. Russell Blaylock, a renowned neurosurgeon, has written numerous papers and books about the neurotoxic effects of aspartame, and suggests an association with multiple sclerosis, epilepsy, Parkinson's disease, Alzheimer's disease, lymphoma, fibromyalgia, and diabetes. We recommend you avoid it.

Saccharin (brand name Sweet'N Low)— made through the chemical reaction of anthranilic acid, nitrous oxide, sulfur dioxide, chlorine (a known carcinogen), and ammonia—was linked to bladder cancer in rats in the 1970s. However, later studies did not provide clear evidence of an association between saccharin and cancer in humans. We think there are better options.

Sucralose (brand name Splenda), a sugar derivative, was discovered in the process of creating pesticides and has been shown to increase HbA_{1c} (your average blood sugar levels). In one study, it was shown to decrease the amount of healthy bacteria in the gut.

SUGAR ALCOHOLS:
THE GOOD, BAD AND UGLY

What are sugar alcohols? They are neither sugar nor alcohol, but they are carbohydrates. Their chemical structure resembles that of half sugar and half alcohol, but they won't get you drunk. Sugar alcohols are an alternative to sugar (used in moderation) for people with insulin resistance and diabetes. But not all sugar alcohols are the same. Some are safer than others and have fewer side effects.

The Good: Sugar alcohols occur naturally in many plants and fruits and are now being widely marketed as sugar substitutes. They are generally a safe sugar substitute. Most look and taste like sugar and are great for baking. Some of them will raise blood sugar and cause the body to release insulin, but much more slowly and not nearly as much as sugar does (except erythritol, which doesn't raise blood sugar or insulin). However, caution should be taken if you have irritable bowel syndrome (IBS). Sugar alcohols should be avoided if you have Crohn's disease or ulcerative colitis.

The Bad: Because sugar alcohols are not technically sugar, manufacturers can misleadingly advertise foods containing them as being sugar free. But sugar alcohols still count as a unique class of carbs, which ultimately count as sugar and can lead to insulin resistance if overconsumed (except for erythritol). When calculating the amount of carbohydrates that these sweeteners contain, take the total carbohydrate count and divide it in half. In other words, the carbohydrates from sugar alcohols count for about half of regular carbs.

The Ugly: The body can't digest sugar alcohols easily, which is why they don't spike insulin quickly. This is good and bad, but can lead to an ugly side effect. Sugar alcohols remain in the gastrointestinal tract much longer than sugar (which is immediately absorbed into the bloodstream). Anything that stays in the gastrointestinal tract for an extended time will ferment. This can cause bloating, gas, stomach pain, and diarrhea in some people, which is why sugar alcohols can be especially problematic for those who have IBS, Crohn's disease, or ulcerative colitis. So we wouldn't suggest consuming a large dessert sweetened with sugar alcohols if you have a special date or are meeting your future in-laws for the first time. The impression you make might not be the one you were hoping for! The two sugar alcohols that most commonly cause digestive problems are maltitol and xylitol, and they are the most commercially used. Erythritol is less likely to be problematic for most people because it is digested differently from maltitol and xylitol.

Not all sugar alcohols affect people the same way or have the same composition. For example, maltitol tends to cause more gastrointestinal distress for many people, and it contains a higher level of carbohydrates than some of the others, so it increases blood sugar more. Xylitol does have a significant calorie and carbohydrate content, but it tends to cause less gastrointestinal distress for many people and inhibits the growth of dental cavities, which is why it is commonly added to sugar-free gum.

Erythritol is our favorite sugar alcohol to use as a sugar substitute. It comes as crystals that resemble sugar or in a powdered form. It has no calories and doesn't spike blood sugar or insulin. While erythritol causes less gastrointestinal distress than most other sugar alcohols, it should still be used with caution until you know how you will react to it. Erythritol is digested in the small intestines, while xylitol and maltitol are digested in the large intestines. The extra time in the gastrointestinal tract allows for more fermentation for xylitol and maltitol, which is the cause of the increased gastrointestinal distress.

STEVIA: A BETTER ALTERNATIVE

The stevia leaf is an herb. Many people refer to it as the natural alternative sweetener. We have a personal bias toward stevia as a sweetener because it has the least reported problems and the greatest reported health claims. However, unless you are crushing stevia leaves and using them to sweeten your favorite drink, we're not talking about a totally natural sweetener. Most people buy stevia extract rather than growing their own plants. Extracted from stevia leaves, which are dried with a water-extraction process, the sweetener is refined using ethanol, methanol, and crystallization. It then goes through ultrafiltration and nanofiltration to remove those alcohols. While this process doesn't technically qualify as natural, the alcohols are removed in the end. Also, there are no other chemicals being combined to *create* stevia.

Stevia extract is as much as 200 to 300 times sweeter than sugar, so you need only the tiniest amount. If you use too much, you may find that it tastes bitter.

Stevia does not impact blood sugar levels the way sugar does. There is some evidence to suggest that it may stabilize blood sugar levels, enhance glucose tolerance, and reduce blood pressure—but more research is needed. If you take blood pressure medication or medication for diabetes, use stevia with caution. There is some evidence that it may act synergistically with these medications and could cause hypotension (low blood pressure) and hypoglycemia (low blood sugar).

Stevia should be used in limited amounts, as it still keeps the taste buds hooked on the sweet taste of foods. Also the message is still being sent to your body that something sweet is coming.

GO AGAINST THE GRAIN

Almost without fail when we do nutrition lectures, explaining the downside of grains, there are several people who raise their hands and quickly point out that Jesus ate bread; therefore, it must be on the approved list of foods. They then proceed to quote scripture. They seem to have a religious attachment to bread! We have great respect for scripture, but large agribusiness was not around making bread for Jesus 2,000 years ago. So what does the wheat from biblical times and the wheat from today have in common? Not much! The genetically hybridized grains of today have little resemblance to the pure wild grains of yesteryear. That's the problem. The human digestive system is not designed to process modern grains as a major staple. Before the advent of farming and agriculture, our hunter-gatherer ancestors had access to only small amounts of *wild* grains and ate them sparingly. But with the agricultural revolution in the early seventeen hundreds grains were eaten in larger amounts. Unfortunately, many grains quickly turn to sugar in your body. When humans started eating grains in large amounts obesity, heart disease, diabetes, and cancer all increased.

At Amen Clinics we find that our best testimonials often come when we put patients on gluten-, dairy-, and sugar-free diets.

From a Patient in Hong Kong

"I have been following the diet since we last spoke. No dairy, gluten, or sugar. How do I feel? Nice and focused. More focused than before and my emotions are in check. The new diet has made a significant positive impact on my mental health. I am indeed very sensitive to what I eat. My moods, my thoughts, feelings and even my behavior and self-control are better. Now that my eyes are open it is really scary to see so much junk food produced commercially. There needs to be more awareness on what exactly is good for us and what is not. Thank God I have no more cravings just like you said. After one week on the new diet I am, surprisingly, very disciplined and positively selective with what I eat. I just laugh at the supermarkets because as far as I'm concerned, more than 70% of what they supply I now consider junk food. From cakes, preserved food, ice cream, chocolates etc. All junk. Thank you so much."

From the Mother of a Patient from Ecuador

"Since coming to the clinic and starting on the diet a year ago, my daughter has lost 70 pounds and has been transformed. Her follow-up SPECT study showed improvement. She has been eating gluten-, dairy-, and sugar-free for the last year and she says the program saved her life."

GLUTEN IS THE GLUE IN GRAINS

The word *gluten* is Latin for "glue." Gluten is a sticky substance found in wheat, barley (and malt, which is made from barley), rye, kamut, bulgur, and spelt. It gives bread dough its elasticity, helps it rise, and gives baked bread its chewy texture. Gluten is found in most commercially made breads, cakes, cookies, cereals, pasta, and many other grain-based products.

Gluten-related health issues are on the rise. Gluten is associated with celiac disease, type 1 diabetes, and Hashimoto's thyroid disease—all of which are autoimmune conditions. Gluten can also trigger flu-like symptoms, psychological disturbances, skin rashes, acne, inflammation, alopecia (baldness), arthritis, and food addiction. Approximately 3 million Americans have celiac disease (formerly known as celiac sprue), a genetic condition in which eating gluten causes an immune reaction that tells the body to attack and destroy villi, the fingerlike structures in the small intestines that absorb nutrients from food. As damaged intestinal villi lose their ability to absorb nutrients there is a diminished capacity for the intestines to absorb essential vitamins and minerals, leading to deficiencies. In babies and children, this can lead to a failure to thrive and grow normally. The number of people with celiac disease has *quadrupled* in the past fifty years. And many experts believe that the number of people with celiac disease is grossly underestimated due to lack of education and poor testing methods.

According to the Center for Celiac Research and Treatment, an additional 18 million Americans have *gluten sensitivity*, which the center recognizes as a serious health issue. Although gluten sensitivity does not qualify as celiac disease, when people who are sensitive to gluten eat foods with gluten, they can experience celiac-like symptoms. Gluten sensitivity can lead to more than a hundred different symptoms that include chronic diarrhea, bloating, flatulence, nausea, abdominal pain, skin rashes, fatigue, and mental fogginess. Many times these symptoms are attributed to other causes and conditions because of the lack of awareness about gluten sensitivity. In our opinion, there is no healthy reason to eat gluten-containing bread, rolls, or pastries. Furthermore, the modified food starch and maltodextrin found in many processed foods are often sourced from gluten as is even the innocuous-sounding ingredient, natural flavor.

GLUTEN: CAUSE FOR CONCERN

- About 40 percent more in bread today than fifty years ago due to hybridization
- Hidden in
  salad dressings
  sauces
  processed foods
  cosmetics
  most cold cut meats, bacon, and sausage
  chicken and turkey (with added solution)
- High glycemic
- May increase inflammation
- Associated with autoimmune issues
- Can increase insulin resistance
- Can cause lower brain blood flow[75]
- Associated with a subset of patients with schizophrenic and mood disorders[76]
- Associated with cerebellar abnormalities, and 40 percent of idiopathic sporadic ataxia[77]

- Associated with intractable seizures and hippocampal atrophy

Gluten-free diets are associated with:
- Reduction, even full remission, of symptoms in subset of schizophrenic patients[78]
- Improvement in autistic and ADHD symptoms in a subset of patients[79]

SOY MANY PROBLEMS!

Contrary to what popular marketing would indicate, soy is not the miracle food perfect for replacing meat and dairy. Although soy can offer some health benefits—when eaten in moderation, in the right form and at the right times—its disadvantages outweigh its advantages, for the most part. One of the problems with soy is that we are inundated with it—commercial salad dressings and other products contain soy oil, many processed foods are manufactured with soy protein isolate, and soy chips claim space next to potato chips and other junk snacks on supermarket shelves. Constant exposure to soy can lead to increased sensitivity to it.

Soy also contains components that are harmful to our health, such as the following:

- A high concentration of lectins (which are more difficult to destroy [with heat] than almost any other lectin-containing food)
- Large amounts of omega-6 fatty acids, which in excessive amounts can lead to systemic inflammation
- Phytoestrogens (plant estrogens) that may or may not contribute to the development of cancer, early puberty in girls, and impotence in men
- A substantial amount of phytic acid, which is believed to reduce the absorption of vital minerals
- More than 80 percent of soy in America is genetically modified, although organic edamame and fermented tofu are the exceptions

BE CAUTIOUS WITH CORN

Corn is referred to as "the king of crops" because of its unparalleled abundance in America. It is also inexpensive, which is why corn derivatives end up in nearly every packaged food. Corn oil, corn syrup, cornstarch, corn alcohol, ethanol, and even corn *gluten* (and many, many more) are now found in nearly all fast foods, processed foods, pesticides, and even toiletry products.

Corn has the most unhealthy fatty acid profile of just about any grain. Being high in omega-6 fatty acids and very low in omega-3 fatty acids makes corn an inflammatory food. It's also a breeding ground for twenty-two different fungi and contains high levels of aspergillus, a type of mold. Like most grains, corn has been shown to damage the intestinal lining, create intestinal permeability, and disrupt blood sugar balance because the *lipid transfer protein* (a protein on the surface of cells in corn) is indigestible by humans. Lipid transfer protein is not broken down during cooking, and it is linked to corn allergies that produce symptoms such as skin rashes, asthma, swelling of mucus membranes, diarrhea, and vomiting. Archaeological records of Native North American and Mayan cultures reveal that when these peoples traded their traditional hunter-gatherer lifestyles for a corn-based diet, they began suffering from malnutrition, osteoporosis, and anemia.

CORN CONCERNS

- Nearly two-thirds of all packaged food contains corn.
- About 85 percent of corn is genetically modified.
- It makes animals *fat* and deposits fat in the muscles.
- Corn gluten meal is a natural herbicide that kills other plants.
- Corn causes celiac-like lesions in intestines by damaging villi.
- It's associated with decreased absorption of vital minerals and nutrients.
- Corn contains twenty-two micotoxins, including aflatoxin and fumonisin.

Corn gluten is actually used as an herbicide to kill certain seeds and herbs. When other plants die they decompose and serve as a fertilizer to nourish other plants. Not corn! To make matters worse, the pollen from corn, which is spread by wind, kills Monarch butterflies (considered a primary species for conservation) and caterpillars that eat affected ragweed nearby.

We are also very concerned about the widespread use of the glyphosate pesticide Roundup, which is sprayed on corn and is banned in some European countries; it has been shown to be one of the most toxic substances to human cells.[80] It is also associated with ADHD,[81] cancer, depression, Parkinson's disease, multiple sclerosis, hypothyroidism, and liver disease.[82]

Although eliminating all corn can be difficult, simply eliminating processed foods and recipes containing corn kernels can radically reduce your exposure.

WHY DO FARMERS FEED ANIMALS CORN, SOY, AND POTATOES?

Farmers feed their animals corn, soy, and potatoes to make them fat quickly!

We were in Washington, D.C., a number of years ago speaking at a conference. Afterward, we took Chloe to George Washington's plantation at Mount Vernon. While strolling around the grounds we came across a plaque that read: HOGS.

Pork was a source of food for virtually every member of the Mount Vernon community. Bacon, ham, and lard were most often consumed. Difficult to keep penned, the hogs generally ran loose in the woods. In the late fall they were captured, *fattened on corn and potatoes*, and then slaughtered. That is why we suggest you hold the corn and the potatoes unless you want to wear them on your rear.

MILK IS FOR BABY COWS, NOT YOU

Unless you grew up on another planet, you've heard that milk "does a body good." Advertising has told you that if you haven't "got milk" you're missing out on something. And you've seen a constellation of movie stars and celebrities smiling at you from beneath their milk mustaches in the pages of glossy magazines. All of these advertising tricks are an attempt to get you to consume a food that your body doesn't need—a food that does a body way more harm than good.

Top nutrition scientists are beginning to recognize what many human intestines have already made clear: Cow's milk is unnecessary in the human diet. Mammals are not designed to drink milk past infancy, and during infancy they should be drinking milk from their own mother, not a lactating animal from another species. Many humans have trouble digesting dairy products. After the age of two, fewer than 35 percent of humans produce the enzyme lactase, which is needed to break down lactose (milk sugar) and digest milk. People of Jewish, Italian, West African, Arab, Greek, and Asian descent are among those least likely to produce lactase. Without lactase in your gut, lactose remains undigested, fermenting in your intestines and causing an array of gastrointestinal symptoms referred to as lactose intolerance. It would really be more accurate to call the few who can easily digest cow's milk "lactase persistent," because the inability to tolerate lactose is actually the norm. Even if your body can break down lactose, it's still bad news because it is converted to galactose and glucose, which elevate blood sugar and can cause inflammation.

Also, casein (a protein in milk) is an excitotoxin in the brain. Left unchecked, excitotoxins lead to brain inflammation and neurodegenerative diseases. Casein has also been shown to bind to polyphenols found in coffee, tea, berries, and vegetables, rendering these potent nutrients useless.

But what about calcium? Don't you need calcium from milk to keep your bones strong and ward off osteoporosis? The answer is yes, you do need calcium. But you are better off getting calcium from plants. The calcium in milk is not easily utilized by the body, and there's no solid proof that it improves bone strength or prevents bone thinning and osteoporosis. Research with non-milk-drinking Asians has found they get all the calcium they need from plant foods. Osteoporosis rates are much lower in milk-free Asians than in milk-addicted Americans. Green leafy vegetables, exercise, and increased protein intake are more effective ways for your body to get the calcium it needs. And, unlike these ways of getting calcium, milk doesn't promote weight loss or reduce the risk of cardiovascular disease either. In fact, dairy products are actually associated with an increased risk of acne, prostate cancer, Parkinson's disease, and joint pain.

Here are some more reasons to limit milk:

- Pasteurization—the process of heating milk to a high temperature for a short time to kill bacteria—also kills most of the live enzymes that may have made milk slightly worth drinking. While pasteurization is necessary to prevent food poisoning, it renders milk relatively useless, nutritionally speaking. Organic milk is even worse than conventionally produced milk because it requires ultrapasteurization, which kills even more enzymes.
- Homogenization, the process of breaking up the fat in milk so it won't separate, may also break down a substance in the milk called plasminogen, which may elevate the risk of arteriosclerosis.
- Bovine growth hormones rBST and rBGH are commonly given to dairy cows to increase their milk production. Their presence in the milk you drink stimulates your liver to produce insulin growth factor 1 (IGF-1). Milk already contains significant amounts of IGF-1, but the addition of these hormones causes your body to produce even more. Excessive IGF-1 has been associated with tumor promoters for breast and prostate cancer. Prostate cancer has been linked to dairy products in several studies. In the Harvard Physicians' Health Study, which included more than 20,000 male physicians, those who consumed more than two dairy servings daily had a 34 percent higher risk of developing prostate cancer than men who consumed few or no dairy products.[83]
- Natural estrogens from pregnant cows can increase the risk of hormone-sensitive cancers, such as prostate, testicular, and breast,[84] and are suspected of contributing to early puberty in our children.
- The rBGH given to cows makes them more susceptible to infection, especially mastitis. Infections are treated with antibiotics, which find their way into the milk you drink. Overuse of antibiotics can also lead to the growth of antibiotic-resistant bacteria. Many countries have banned milk from cows that have been treated with rBGH.
- In several studies, there is a link between drinking milk and Parkinson's disease, which may be due to pesticide exposure.[85]

PLAIN YOGURT AND CLARIFIED BUTTER

While we are not fans of most dairy products, for the reasons just discussed, plain yogurt and clarified butter may have a place in a Brain Warrior's diet. We are not talking about flavored yogurts loaded with sugar (read the labels), but *plain* yogurt that boosts protein and probiotics. If you eat plain yogurt, add frozen berries and a little stevia to make it taste great.

Clarified butter or ghee may be useful because it has short-chain fatty acids that have been shown to be helpful in gut healing. The milk proteins casein and whey have been removed, so people tend to have fewer allergies to it.

GOAT'S MILK IS A GOOD ALTERNATIVE

- More calcium and magnesium than cow's milk
- It has more protein than cow's milk.
- About 93 percent of infants with milk allergies can drink goat's milk.
- Goat's milk is naturally homogenized.
- It is easier to digest.
- Goats are not typically given hormones and antibiotics.
- It still contains lactose.

WHAT IF CHEESE IS MY CRACK?

If you think about cheese constantly you may be addicted to it. A new study suggests addiction to dairy is a real thing.[86] It examined why certain foods are more addictive than others. The researchers identified addictive foods from about 500 people who completed the Yale Food Addiction Scale, designed to measure if someone has a food addiction. Pizza, it may not be surprising, came out on top of the most-addictive-food list. Besides being a basic food group for kids, college students, and adults, there's a scientific reason we all love pizza, and it has to do with the cheese. The study found certain foods are addictive because of the way they are processed. The more processed and fatty the food, the more it was associated with addictive eating behaviors. Cheese happens to be especially addictive because when the dairy protein casein is combined with stomach acid it produces casomorphins, which have a mild opiate- or heroin-like effect in the brain. Bet you can't eat just one slice of pizza? When Daniel used to go to his parents' house for Christmas his mom made amazing pizza. Even though he always promised himself he wouldn't eat more than two slices, he would often have eight slices. Casomorphins trump willpower. Now he goes there after he has eaten a healthy meal and might have one slice.

ADDICTIVE QUALITIES OF GLUTEN AND CHEESE

- When gluten and casein are exposed to pepsin and hydrochloric acid in the stomach they break down to exorphins, which cross the blood–brain barrier.
- These bind to endorphin (morphinelike) receptors and can cause a mild euphoria.
- This effect is blocked by naltrexone, the medicine that blocks the effect of morphine and heroin in the brain.
- Many people have withdrawal symptoms when they stop gluten or dairy.
- Binge eaters eat less (especially wheat) when given naltrexone.

Now that you know more about the foods to choose and the foods to lose and why, it will be easier for you to make better decisions about what to eat. We often say, "Know better, do better." In Part 7 we put all of this information together for you in the 14-Day Brain Boosting Plan.

SUPPLEMENT YOUR SUCCESS

Using supplements by themselves, without getting your diet, exercise, thoughts, peer group, and environment under control, is a waste of money. You need to embrace the whole program for it to work. We have seen that when supplements are used in conjunction with the Brain Warrior's Way program, they can make a significant difference.

There are pros and cons to using natural supplements to enhance brain function. To start, they are often effective. They usually have dramatically fewer side effects than most prescription medications and they are significantly less expensive. Plus you never have to tell an insurance company that you have taken them. As awful as it sounds, taking prescription medications can affect your insurability. We know many people who have been denied or made to pay higher rates for life, health, disability, or long-term-care insurance because they have taken certain medications. If there are natural alternatives, they are worth considering.

Yet natural supplements also have their own set of problems. For instance, even though they tend to be less expensive than medications, they may cost more out-of-pocket because they are usually not covered by insurance. Also, many people are unaware that natural supplements can have side effects and need to be thoughtfully used. Just because something is natural does not mean it is innocuous. Both arsenic and cyanide are natural, but that doesn't mean they are good for you. For example, St. John's Wort, one of our favorite natural antidepressants, can cause sun sensitivity and it can also decrease the effectiveness of a number of medications such as birth control pills.

One of the major concerns about natural supplements is the lack of quality control. There is a lot of variability and you need to find brands you trust. Make sure any supplements you buy are from manufacturers that follow the good manufacturing practices (GMP) developed by the FDA. Another pitfall is that many people get their advice about supplements from the clerks at health food stores who may not have the best information. But even when looking at the problems, the benefits of natural supplements make them worth considering, especially if you can get thoughtful, research-based information. Every day we each take a handful of supplements that we believe make a significant difference in our lives.

Many physicians say that if you eat a balanced diet you do not need supplements. We appreciate what Mark Hyman wrote in his book *The UltraMind Solution: Fix Your Broken Brain by Healing Your Body First*. He wrote that if people "eat wild, fresh, organic, local, nongenetically modified food grown in virgin mineral- and nutrient-rich soils that has not been transported across vast distances and stored for months before being eaten . . . and work and live outside, breathe only fresh unpolluted air, drink only pure, clean water, sleep nine hours a night, move their bodies every day, and are free from chronic stressors and exposure to environmental toxins," then it is possible that they might not need supplements.[87] However, because people live in a fast-paced society where they pick up food on the fly, skip meals, eat sugar-laden treats, buy processed foods, and eat foods that have been chemically treated, most people could use a little help from a multiple vitamin/mineral supplement.

Research demonstrates the therapeutic benefits of using supplements to support a healthy mood, sleep, and memory. When purchasing a supplement, we strongly recommend that you consult a health-care practitioner familiar with nutritional supplements to determine which supplements and dosages may be most effective for you. Our website (brainmdhealth.com) contains links to the scientific literature on many different supplements related to brain health, so you, as a consumer, can be fully informed on the benefits and risks involved. Please remember supplements can have very powerful effects on the body and caution should be used when combining them with prescription medications.

THREE ESSENTIAL SUPPLEMENTS FOR EVERYONE

There are three supplements we typically recommend to all of our patients because they are critical to optimal brain function: a multivitamin, omega-3 fatty acids, and vitamin D.

Multivitamin

According to recent studies, more than 50 percent of Americans do not eat at least five servings of fruits and vegetables a day—the minimum required to get the nutrition you need. We recommend that all of our patients take a high-quality multivitamin/mineral complex every day. In an editorial in the *Journal of the American Medical Association*, researchers recommended a daily vitamin for everybody because it helps prevent chronic illness. In addition, people with weight-management issues often are not eating healthy diets and have vitamin and nutrient deficiencies. Plus research suggests that people who take a multiple vitamin actually have younger-looking DNA.

A 2010 study from Northumbria University[88] tested the effects of multivitamins on 215 men between the ages of thirty and fifty-five. For the double-blind, placebo-controlled study, the men were assessed on mental performance and asked to rate themselves on general mental health, stress, and mood. At the debut of the trial, there were no significant differences between the multivitamin group and the placebo group. When the participants were retested a little over one month later, the multivitamin group reported improved moods and showed better mental performance, helping them be happier and smarter! Not only that, but the multivitamin group reported an improved sense of vigor, reduced stress, and less mental fatigue after completing mental tasks.

In another placebo-controlled study from Northumbria,[89] researchers tested the effects of multivitamins on eighty-one healthy children from ages eight to fourteen. They found that the children who took multivitamins performed better on two out of three attention tasks. The researchers concluded that multivitamins have the potential to improve brain function in healthy children.

Omega-3 Fatty Acids

For years, we have been writing about the benefits of omega-3 fatty acids, which are found in fish oil supplements. Personally, we both take omega-3 fatty acids every day and recommend all of our patients do the same. When you see the mountain of scientific evidence, it is easy to understand why. Research has found that omega-3 fatty acids are essential for optimal brain and body health.

For example, according to researchers at the Harvard School of Public Health, having low levels of omega-3 fatty acids is one of the leading preventable causes of death and has been associated with heart disease, strokes, depression, suicidal behavior, ADD, dementia, and obesity. There is also scientific evidence that low levels of omega-3 fatty acids play a role in substance abuse.

Unless focusing on eating fish or taking fish oil supplements, most people have low omega-3 levels. We know this because at the Amen Clinics we perform a blood test on patients to measure the levels of omega-3 fatty acids in the blood. Before we began offering the test to patients, we tested it on our employees, several family members, and of course, ourselves. When Daniel's test results came back, he was very happy with the robust numbers. An omega-3 score above seven is good. His was nearly eleven. But the results for nearly all of the employees and family members tested were not so good, which put them at greater risk for both physical and emotional problems. It is an easy fix. They just needed to eat more fish or take fish oil supplements.

Boosting your intake of omega-3 fatty acids is one of the best things you can do for your brainpower, mood, and weight. The two most studied omega-3 fatty acids are EPA and DHA. DHA makes up a large portion of the gray matter of the brain. The fat in your brain forms cell membranes and plays a vital role in how our cells function. Neurons are also rich in omega-3 fatty acids. EPA improves blood flow, which boosts overall brain function.

Increasing omega-3 intake has been found to decrease appetite and cravings and reduce body fat. In a fascinating 2009 study in the *British Journal of Nutrition*,[90] Australian researchers analyzed blood samples, calculated BMIs, and measured waist and hip circumferences for 124 adults (21 healthy weight, 40 overweight, and 63 obese). They found that obese individuals had significantly lower levels of EPA and DHA compared with healthy-weight people. Subjects with higher levels were more likely to have a healthy BMI and waist and hip measurements.

More evidence about the benefits of fish oil on weight loss comes from a 2007 study from the University of South Australia.[91] The research team found that taking fish oil combined with moderate exercise, such as walking for 45 minutes three times a week, leads to a significant reduction in body fat after just twelve weeks. But taking fish oil without exercising, or exercising without fish oil, did not result in any reduction in body fat.

One of the most intriguing studies on fish oil and weight loss appeared in a 2007 issue of the *International Journal of Obesity*.[92] In this study, researchers from Iceland investigated the effects of seafood and fish oils on weight loss in 324 young overweight men with BMI ranging from 27.5 to 32.5. The participants were placed in four groups; each ate the same 1,600-calorie diet except for the addition of only one of the following:

- Control group (sunflower oil capsules, no seafood or fish oil)
- Lean fish (three 150-gram portions of cod per week)
- Fatty fish (three 150-gram portions of salmon per week)
- Fish oil (DHA/EPA capsules, no seafood)

After four weeks, the average amount of weight loss among the men in each of the four groups was as follows:

- Control group: 7.8 pounds
- Lean fish group: 9.6 pounds
- Fatty fish group: 9.9 pounds
- Fish oil group: 10.9 pounds

The researchers concluded that adding fish or fish oil to a nutritionally balanced, calorie-restricted diet could boost weight loss in men.

Research in the last few years has also revealed that diets rich in omega-3 fatty acids help promote a healthy emotional balance and positive mood in later years, possibly because DHA is a main component of the brain's synapses. A growing body of scientific evidence indicates that fish oil helps ease symptoms of depression. One twenty-year study involving 3,317 men and women found that people with the highest consumption of EPA and DHA were less likely to have symptoms of depression.

There is a tremendous amount of scientific evidence pointing to a connection between the consumption of fish that is rich in omega-3 fatty acids and cognitive function. A Danish team of researchers compared the diets of 5,386 healthy older individuals and found that the more fish in a person's diet, the longer the person was able to maintain their memory and reduce the risk of dementia. J. A. Conquer and colleagues from the University of Guelph in Guelph, Ontario, Canada, studied the blood fatty acid content in the early and later stages of dementia and noted low levels when compared to healthy people. In 2010, UCLA researchers analyzed the existing scientific literature on DHA and fish oil and concluded that supplementation with DHA slows the progression of Alzheimer's disease and may prevent age-related dementia.

Omega-3 fatty acids may benefit cognitive performance and behavior at every age. Scientists at the University of Pittsburgh reported in 2010 that middle-aged people with higher DHA levels performed better on a variety of tests, including nonverbal reasoning, mental flexibility, working memory, and vocabulary.[93] Swedish researchers who surveyed nearly 5,000 fifteen-year-old boys found that those who ate fish more than once a week scored higher on standard intelligence tests than teens who ate no fish.[94] A follow-up study found that teens eating fish more than once a week also had better grades at school than students with lower fish consumption.[95] A 2015 placebo-controlled study showed that 1 gram per day of omega-3 fatty acids in eight- to sixteen-year-olds significantly improved their behavior.[96]

Additional benefits of omega-3 fatty acids include increased attention in people with ADD, reduced stress, and a lower risk for psychosis. When we put our retired football players on our fish oil supplements, many of them were able to decrease or completely eliminate their pain medications.

Our recommendation for most adults is to take between 1 and 2 grams per day of high-quality fish oil that is balanced between EPA and DHA.

Vitamin D

Vitamin D, also known as the "sunshine vitamin," is best known for building bones and boosting the immune system. But it is also an essential vitamin for brain health, mood, memory, and weight. While classified as a vitamin, it is actually a steroid hormone vital to health. Low levels of vitamin D have been associated with depression, autism, psychosis, Alzheimer's disease, multiple sclerosis, heart disease, diabetes, cancer, and obesity. Unfortunately, vitamin D deficiencies are becoming more and more common, in part because we are spending more time indoors and using more sunscreen. While the latter is necessary to protect your skin from damage, it also blocks the body's ability to synthesize vitamin D from sunlight.

Did you know that when you don't have enough vitamin D, you feel hungry all the time, no matter how much you eat? This is because low levels of vitamin D interfere with the effectiveness of leptin, the appetite hormone that tells you when you are full. Research also shows that vitamin D deficiency is associated with increased body fat. A 2009 study out of Canada found that weight and body fat were significantly lower in women with normal vitamin D levels than in women with insufficient levels.[97] It appears that extra fat inhibits the absorption of vitamin D. The evidence shows that obese people need higher doses of vitamin D than lean people do to achieve the same levels.

One of the most interesting studies on vitamin D comes from researchers at Stanford Health Care. Researchers detailed how a patient was given a prescription for 50,000 IU weekly of vitamin D that was incorrectly filled for 50,000 IU daily instead of weekly. After six months, the patient's vitamin D level increased from 7, which is extremely low, to 100, which is at the high end of normal.

What we found really intriguing about this report was that the patient complained of a few side effects from the very high dosage, namely decreased appetite and significant weight loss. Of course, we are not advocating that you take more vitamin D than you need because it can be toxic, but it indicates that optimal levels of vitamin D may play a role in appetite control and weight loss. This patient's story shows why it is so important to get your vitamin D level checked before and after treatment. That way, you will know if you are taking the right dosage.

Vitamin D is so important to brain function that its receptors can be found throughout the brain. Vitamin D plays a critical role in many of the most basic cognitive functions, including learning and making memories. These are just some of the areas where vitamin D affects how well your brain works.[98]

The scientific community is waking up to the importance of vitamin D for optimal brain function. In the past few years, there have been a number of studies linking a shortage of vitamin D with cognitive impairment in older men and women as well as some suggesting that having optimal levels of the sunshine vitamin may play a role in protecting cognitive function. One such study in the *Journal of Alzheimer's Disease* found that vitamin D$_3$, the active form of vitamin D, may stimulate the immune system to rid the brain of beta amyloid,[99] an abnormal protein that is believed to be a major cause of Alzheimer's disease. Vitamin D activates receptors on neurons in regions important in the regulation of behavior, and it protects the brain by acting in an antioxidant and anti-inflammatory capacity.

Another study conducted in 2009 by a team at Tufts University in Boston looked at vitamin D levels in more than 1,000 people over the age of sixty-five and its effect on cognitive function. Only 35 percent of the participants had optimal vitamin D levels; the rest fell in the insufficient or deficient categories. The individuals with optimal levels of vitamin D (50 nmol/L or higher) performed better on tests of executive functions, such as reasoning, flexibility, and perceptual complexity. They also scored higher on attention and processing-speed tests than their counterparts with suboptimal levels.[100]

The lower your vitamin D levels, the more likely you are to feel down rather than happy. Low levels of vitamin D have long been associated with a higher incidence of depression. In recent years, researchers have been asking if, given this association, vitamin D supplementation can improve moods.

One trial that attempted to answer this question followed 441 overweight and obese adults with similar levels of depression for one year. The individuals took either a placebo or one or two doses of vitamin D: 20,000 IU per week or 40,000 IU per week. By year's end, the two groups that had taken the vitamin D showed a significant reduction in symptoms while the group taking the placebo reported no improvements.[101] Other trials have reported similar findings.

The current recommended dose for vitamin D is 400 IU daily, but most experts agree that this is well below the physiological needs of most individuals and instead suggest 2,000 IU of vitamin D daily. We think it is very important to test your individual needs, especially if you are overweight or obese because your body may not absorb the vitamin D as efficiently as it should when you are heavier.

We also recommend you take probiotics and other multiple-mechanism supplements discussed in Part 2 as well as those targeted to your unique brain type.

BRAIN WARRIOR MOTHER ANGELA

"After my daughter was born she constantly threw up and would scream bloody murder. I was told she had a milk allergy and acid reflux and she was placed on medication. It was a nonstop struggle. At two years old, she was extremely emotional and would have severe mood swings and angry outbursts. This continued on and on. One night my mother couldn't sleep and watched one of your public television shows and told me to watch it too. I subsequently ordered 2 books and a video. In 2013, when my daughter was 7, we had an evaluation and scans done at your Virginia clinic. On a gluten- and dairy-free diet, plus a probiotic and several supplements my daughter is a changed child. She went from constant turmoil, endless battles with schools, and not being able to attend regular classes, to a healthy 9-year-old who attends regular class. Thank you for giving my daughter her smile back."

Brain Warrior Sustenance Takeaways

SUMMARY OF THE TEN BRAIN WARRIOR NUTRITION PRINCIPLES

1. Focus on high-quality calories.
2. Drink plenty of water and not many of your calories.
3. Eat high-quality protein in small doses throughout the day.
4. Eat smart carbohydrates (low glycemic, high fiber).
5. Focus your diet on healthy fats.
6. Eat from the rainbow, which means healthful foods of many different colors (not Skittles!).
7. Cook with brain healthy herbs and spices to boost your brain and body.
8. Make sure your food is as clean as possible: organic, hormone free, antibiotic free, grass fed, and free range.
9. If you struggle with any mental health or physical issue, eliminate any potential allergens or internal attackers, such as MSG, gluten, corn, soy, and dairy.
10. Eat healthfully during the day, but fast for 12 hours at night.

FOODS TO CHOOSE

100 Best Brain Healthy Foods

FOODS TO LOSE

- Sugar
- Eat grains like you would condiments
- Gluten
- Soy
- Corn
- Dairy

SUPPLEMENT YOUR SUCCESS

- Three supplements for everybody
- Multiple-mechanism approach
- Target supplements to your brain type

PART 4

Training of a Brain Warrior

The Daily Habits and Routines for Ultimate Success

When the training is hard, the battle is easy. Warriors don't wait until fight day to start training. *They train every day!*

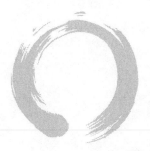

BRAIN WARRIOR NANCY

Nancy came to our clinic from Oxford, England. Three years earlier at the age of eighty, she bought a copy of *Change Your Brain, Change Your Life* in a used bookstore for 50 cents. In her own words, "The book just laid around for a year or two, but when I picked it up I couldn't put it down. It was the most revealing, startling read I think I ever had. Up to that time I had been obese, prone to depression with long low periods, unmotivated, uninspired, and had arthritis. Then I began by thinking about what were the things I could change easily. Little by little I added some of the things recommended."

First, she started to drink more water. By reading the book she learned that her brain is 80 percent water, and staying hydrated was an important brain exercise. After a few days she noticed her energy improved.

Next, she started to take brain healthy supplements, including a multiple vitamin, omega-3 fatty acids, vitamin D (her level tested low), ginkgo biloba, acetyl-L-carnitine, and phosphatidylserine. "They made a big difference," she said.

As her energy increased she began to exercise more, including walking, which helped her mood, and she started to dance and play table tennis.

Motivated by her progress, she completely changed her diet to one just like the Brain Warrior's Way diet described in the last chapter. She became serious about her food and noticed the weight begin to drop away. "I started by eating the good things first, so I lost my cravings for the things that were not good. There was less room for the trash [bad food] in my body."

New learning was her next strategy. She started taking French classes and learned to play the guitar. When we met, she was learning three different languages.

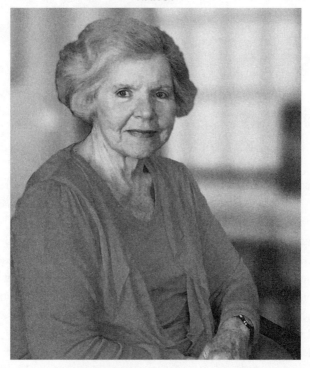

"My life totally changed," she said. "My energy, mood, and memory are remarkably better and I am pain free."

Then she started teaching her family how to love and care for their brains. When they saw their mother get off the couch and shed her weight and depression, they felt it was important to pay attention to what was happening. She said, "The best thing I can do for my children is keep myself healthy for as long as I can. I never dreamt that I could be this happy and have so much fun at this time in my life."

When we met Nancy she had saved her money to come to our clinic in Costa Mesa, California, and get an evaluation including a brain scan. It was her eighty-third-birthday present to herself. After hearing Nancy's inspiring story, our staff invited us to meet her; and when we talked with her, both of us were so moved by her story we started to cry. Nancy is the reason we do what we do. She was so sweet, so grateful, and so funny. She told us she had lost 5 stones.

"How much is that?" Daniel asked.

"Seventy pounds, without counting calories, without depriving my-self of anything I wanted," Nancy replied. "I used to be like this [she made a face like a blowfish]; now I am not. I am off the couch and feeling better than I have in forty years."

Nancy's SPECT scan looked stunningly beautiful. It looked like the brain of a much younger person. She cried when she saw it and said she knew it didn't look anything like that just three years earlier. You are not stuck with the brain you have; you can make it better, no matter when you start.

The main reason for Nancy's success was that she was serious—even relentless—for her brain health. She never felt deprived or had the feeling that her new way of living was hard. Being a couch potato was hard. Being depressed was hard. Feeling isolated and alone was hard. Through the process, she developed the daily habits and routines that propelled her success forward.

In this chapter, we will discuss the daily habits and routines that ensure success with the Brain Warrior's Way. Like Nancy, it is okay to start with just one thing until you master it, and then move on to the next habit.

DAILY HABITS AND ROUTINES OF A BRAIN WARRIOR

So far, this book has taught you about the importance of having a Brain Warrior's mind-set to stay focused and aware, the necessity of assessment and prevention to monitor where you are relative to where you want to go, and the ten vital nutrition principles that are necessary for optimal brain and body function. To further build on your foundation and instill positive discipline into your life, this section is all about training and will teach you the seven daily habits and routines of Brain Warriors that help strengthen your mind and body.

1. Start each day with intention, gratitude, and appreciation.
2. Engage in smart exercise.
3. Flex the muscles between your ears.
4. Combat stress with accelerated mindfulness.
5. Make sleep a priority.
6. Protect your decision-making skills.
7. Be curious, not furious. Become masterful at learning from your mistakes.

1.

Start Each Day with Intention, Gratitude, and Appreciation

Without the vision of a goal, a man cannot manage his life or the lives of others.

—GENGHIS KHAN

Rather than grabbing your phone or laptop as soon as you open your eyes, take 7 minutes to supercharge your brain and start each day in a powerful state of mind. Whatever you visualize, your brain will make it happen. In a world filled with stress, assaults, and unhealthy choices, Brain Warriors are at their best when they start each day by taking a few minutes to breathe deeply and focus their intention, especially on gratitude, appreciation, health, and productivity. Your brain drives your behavior, but you must tell it what you want or it will go with its habitual and deeply programmed behaviors, which are not likely to be in your best interest.

As soon as you open your eyes, read your One Page Miracle (OPM). This is an exercise we encourage our patients and clients to do. Here's how it works: Specify exactly what you want (not what you *don't* want) in the major areas of your life, such as relationships, work, money, and self (physical, emotional, and spiritual health). You can fill out a form online in the Brain Fit Life program (mybrainfitlife.com) or you can write out your OPM on paper. Spend time with developing your One Page Miracle and revise it often. As you read it, ask yourself, "Is *my* behavior getting me what I want?" This will help you focus your thoughts and actions on your goals throughout the day.

It is called the One Page Miracle because it uses two powerful concepts—intention and vision—to tell your brain what you want, so your unconscious mind can help you make it happen. In our experience, when people know what they really want, and continually ask themselves each morning, "Is *my* behavior getting me what I want?" they become more conscientious and effective at making the decisions that serve their health and success rather than making bad decisions that diminish their dreams. The reason *my* is in italics is that it keeps you from blaming other people for how your life is turning out. Whenever you blame your spouse, kids, boss, or society, you become a victim who cannot change anything. You become powerless—the opposite of a warrior. Victims can never win, because their destiny is in someone else's hands. But when you ask yourself, "Is *my* behavior getting me what I want?" you are much more likely to own the problem and solve it. This does not mean you blame yourself; it means you take responsibility for your life. Responsibility is your ability to respond to whatever situation you are in. Reading your OPM first thing in the morning takes only about a minute, but it may be the most powerful minute of the day.

BRAIN WARRIOR MARY

Tana's mother, Mary, was a sixteen-year-old runaway who grew up in poverty and chaos. Her early-childhood memories were of working in the potato sheds and fields to help pay for her own clothes and earn lunch money. As a young child, Mary's mother was taken, screaming, in an ambulance to Camarillo State Mental Hospital. Her father was later in a train accident that left him a quadriplegic. Mary's younger brother struggled to cope and turned to drugs, and her older brother was tragically murdered. In spite of all of this, Mary isn't a survivor; she's a *warrior*!

To say life was hard for Mary and Tana in the early years of Tana's life would be an understatement. Mary was a single working mother who often held three jobs to make ends meet. Women couldn't work more than 8 hours of overtime and, without a high school education, Mary had a hard time finding well-paying jobs. Tana was a latch-key kid and hated not having her mother home. Mary would try to comfort her by painting a picture of her dreams for Tana's future. Mary explained it would require a lot of hard work to get from where they were to where they wanted to go.

One day, a friend of Mary's who lacked ambition saw Mary exhausted and run-down. With a cigarette hanging out of her mouth she said, "You need to stop working so hard. You should just go on government assistance and stay home with your kid." Mary noticed nine-year-old Tana in the corner, listening, and correctly assumed that she thought this would be a great idea—anything to have her mom home more. Choosing her words carefully she said, "I will never allow the government or anyone to have that much control over my life or my destiny. I *know* my hard work will pay off. This is temporary. Taking the easy way out will lead to long-term suffering, and we will be stuck in this hellhole forever. If I act like a victim and give up now I will never win because victims can't win. Someone else controls them."

That was a conversation that would stay with Tana for the rest of her life. It taught her never to be a victim. By the way, Mary has owned a very successful company for the past thirty years (she started in her garage). Her income is now in the top 1 percent of the nation.

After reading your OPM, take another minute or two to write down three things you are grateful for each day. Research has shown that people who do this simple exercise notice a significant increase in their level of happiness in just three weeks. Appreciation is even more powerful than gratitude. Gratitude is an internal state, whereas appreciation is gratitude expressed outwardly by building bridges of positive energy between yourself and others. Once you get your day started, reach out to at least one person and tell her why you appreciate her (do not repeat the same person for at least thirty days). The appreciation exercise will take only another minute or two and supercharges the positive energy in your brain.

2.

Engage in Smart Exercise

> If we could give every individual the right amount of
> nourishment and exercise, not too little and not too much,
> we would have found the safest way to health.
>
> —HIPPOCRATES

If your doctor offered you a prescription that would help you lose weight, lower your risk of numerous life-threatening diseases, boost your energy, make you look and feel sexier, and possibly even help you live longer, you'd most likely rush to a pharmacy to have it filled immediately. There is no such drug. But there is such a treatment! There actually is something you can do that will improve your health in just about every way possible without any worrisome side effects: Engage in moderate exercise on a regular basis. This is no exaggeration. Exercise can do so much for your body that it's kind of mind-boggling that anyone would choose *not* to exercise. Our bodies are designed for *movement*!

One of the most exciting and immediate benefits of exercise is the energy it gives you. One of the women in Tana's classes e-mailed her after a Zumba workout (an exhilarating dance-fitness class set to pulsating Latin and international music), raving: "I came home last night with so much energy and woke up with lots of energy! I have a whole new perspective now since I know what's going on with my body!"

Research has shown that cognitive abilities are best in those who exercise.[102] Exercise improves the flow of oxygen, blood, and nutrients to the brain and protects the brain against things that hurt it, such as high sugar levels. It reduces stress, improves your mood, and lowers your blood pressure and blood sugar levels. Exercise decreases inflammation, fat cells, weight, and frailty, while at the same time increases metabolism, longevity, bone density, and an overall sense of well-being. Research has also shown that regular exercise helps turn off the obesity gene,[103] and positively impacts those at risk for Alzheimer's disease.[104] In addition, exercise has been shown to reduce cravings. One study even found that exercise helps people choose better foods, seek out more social support, and improve sleep.[105]

BETTER THAN ANY PILL

Here are just a few of the benefits of moderate exercise done on a regular basis:

- Improved cognitive abilities
- Improved cognitive flexibility[106]
- Improved mood
- Improved focus
- Improved cardiovascular function
- Slower aging
- Faster loss of body fat and body weight
- Improved lung capacity
- Less inflammation throughout the body
- Lower levels of the stress hormone cortisol
- Higher levels of endorphins and other feel-good neurochemicals

(CONTINUED)

- Higher levels of DHEA, the "fountain of youth" hormone
- Better oxygenation in the body's cells, leading to increased energy and improved cellular health
- Improved insulin sensitivity
- Lower risk of diabetes, heart disease, and some kinds of cancer
- Improved blood pressure
- More muscle mass, which is a protein reserve
- Higher rate of metabolism
- Increased flexibility and agility
- Greater detoxification through sweat
- Better sleep
- Improved ability to stay calm during stressful situations
- Improved immunity

Daily exercise in one form or another is critical to being a Brain Warrior and to your health and longevity. Four types of exercise are great for your brain: bursting or interval training, strength training, coordination exercises, and mindful exercise.[107] Of course, you should check with your physician before starting any new exercise routines.

- **Burst training** involves sixty-second bursts at go-for-broke intensity followed by a few minutes of lower-intensity exertion. We recommend you take a thirty- to forty-five-minute walk every day. During the walk include four or five one-minute periods to "burst" (walk or run as fast as you can), then resume walking at a normal pace. A 2006 study from researchers at the University of Guelph in Canada found that doing high-intensity burst training burns fat faster than continuous moderately intensive activities. Short-burst training helps raise endorphins, lift your mood, and make you feel more energized.
- **Strengthen your brain with strength training.** The stronger you are as you age, the less likely you are to get Alzheimer's disease. Canadian researchers found that resistance training plays a role in preventing cognitive decline.[108] It also helps with weight loss and losing belly fat.[109] We recommend two 30- to 45-minute weight-lifting sessions a week—one for the lower body (abs, lower back, and legs), the other for the upper body (arms, upper back, and chest). A 2010 study from researchers at the University

of Rhode Island compared body composition changes between two groups of dieters.[110] Both groups followed the same nutrition plan, but one group did moderate-intensity resistance training while the other group did not. At the end of the ten-week trial, the group that participated in resistance training lost 9 pounds of body fat compared to less than a half pound for the diet-only group. Plus the resistance training group's thighs got thinner while the other group's thighs remained the same size.

REV YOUR ENGINE

Why should you build muscle and do bursting exercises? Depending on how much muscle you have and how efficiently you train, you could potentially increase your metabolism by ten to fifty times! Think of two cars in freezing weather. The drivers are inside trying to keep the cars warm. One driver just keeps the engine running without ever revving. He's trying to conserve energy. The other driver is constantly hitting the gas pedal and revving the engine, burning through gasoline, even though the car isn't moving.

When you have more muscle and do burst training, which helps train your body to use oxygen, you become like the driver who is revving the engine even though he's sitting still. You burn fuel and energy without doing much, long after your workout. Your metabolism is racing at a higher RPM. The only difference between you and the car is that you will actually have *more* energy as a result because your body will create more of its own fuel. Your cells will produce energy more efficiently when you exercise regularly and intensely.

In addition, muscle is your body's protein reserve in emergencies. Tana witnessed this firsthand as an ICU nurse. Frailty killed elderly patients far faster than disease because it prevented them from recovering and led to increased risk of falls, broken bones, and pneumonia. One study showed that the patients with the most muscle mass had a higher survival rate after serious trauma or burn accidents that required lengthy hospitalization. They also had a better chance of returning to their job and family life without long-term repercussions.

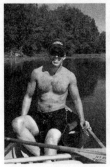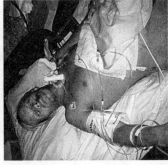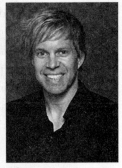

Before · · · · · · · · In Coma · · · · · · · · · · · · · After

Garrett Halweg, one of our psychiatrists, took brain health seriously, including exercise and being strong. While vacationing in Hawaii, he contracted a rare infection called leptospirosis that nearly killed him. He was in a coma for seven days. The only reason he survived, besides the wonderful medical care, was the muscle on his body and the reserve he had built as a result of his daily habits. If he had been frail or even normal, it is likely he would have died. Your life depends on your habits. Because Garrett took brain health seriously, he can continue doing the work he loves that helps so many people.

- **Boost your brain with coordination activities.** Doing coordination activities—like dancing, tennis, or table tennis (the world's best brain sport)—boosts the activity in the cerebellum. While the cerebellum is only 10 percent of the brain's volume, it contains 50 percent of the brain's neurons. It's involved with both physical and thought coordination.
- **Calm and focus your mind with mindful exercise.** Yoga, tai chi, and other mindful exercises have been found to reduce anxiety and depression and increase focus.[111] Although they don't generate the same benefits as aerobic activity, these types of exercises can still boost your brain.
- **Do not overdo it.** High-intensity exercise over a long period of time may be associated with cardiac remodeling and increased risk of cardiovascular problems, such as heart arrhythmias.[112] In a twelve-year follow-up study of twenty high-intensity endurance athletes, 50 percent had enlarged left ventricle walls in the heart, which may not be healthy.[113] This is one area in which we believe

in moderation. Extreme exercise is not necessary to reap the many benefits of exercise—in fact, research suggests that long bouts of highly intensive exercise may actually cause more harm than good. Extreme exercisers often find themselves suffering from the same problems extreme nonexercisers suffer from. Extreme exercise increases oxidative stress and can damage your body. Women who overexercise commonly have amenorrhea (absence of the menstrual period), a result of having very low body fat. Extreme exercise increases the stress hormone cortisol, disrupts neurotransmitter balance (dopamine, serotonin, and glutamine), and alters healthy immune function. The result can be increased inflammation, chronic fatigue, hypothyroidism, altered sleep patterns, increased risk of autoimmune disorders, and physical injury to muscles, bones, and joints. Plus neither of us believes in suffering. Getting well is about smart choices.

One of our close friends was an endurance athlete. He loved running marathons, but also loved ice cream. He told his fiancée that from a dietary perspective he was the exception to the rule and because he exercised so much he could eat like crap and still live to 120 years old. He died in his sleep at the age of fifty-six.

Do all the components of the Brain Warrior's Way if you want to live a long time.

3.

Flex the Muscles Between Your Ears

The more you use your brain, the more you can continue using it. New learning creates new connections in the brain, but the absence of learning causes the brain to start disconnecting itself. Regardless of your age, mental exercise has a global, positive effect on the brain. Learning has a very real impact on neurons: It keeps them firing and it makes it easier for them to fire. There are approximately a thousand trillion synapses in the brain, and each one of them may wither and die if not actively firing. Like muscles that don't get used, idle nerve cells waste away.

Community-dwelling seniors who took five to six weeks of cognitive training that included at least eight 60- to 75-minute training sessions experienced significantly improved reasoning and speed of processing skills, as well as better activities in daily living ten years later, compared with those who didn't get such training, reported a study from Johns Hopkins University.[114]

The best mental exercise is acquiring new knowledge and doing things that you have not done before. Even if your routine activities are fairly complicated, such as teaching a college course, reading brain scans, or fixing a crashed computer network, they won't help your brain specifically because they aren't new to you. Whenever the brain does something over and over, it learns how to do it using less and less energy. New learning, such as learning a new medical technique, a new hobby, or a new game, helps establish new connections, thus maintaining and improving the function of other less-often-used brain areas.[115]

The following list describes which mental exercises provide the best benefits to specific areas of the brain

- Prefrontal cortex (PFC): language games, such as Scrabble, Boggle, Words with Friends, and crossword puzzles; strategy games, such as chess, Rail Baron, Axis, and Blokus; meditation
- Temporal lobes: memory games and learning to play a new musical instrument (also involves PFC and cerebellum)
- Parietal lobes: math games like Sudoku, juggling (also involves PFC and cerebellum), and reading maps
- Cerebellum: coordination games, like table tennis (also involves PFC), dancing (learn new dance steps), yoga, and tai chi

NEW LEARNING TIPS

- Spend fifteen minutes a day learning something new. Einstein said that if anyone spends fifteen minutes a day learning something new, in a year he or she will be an expert; in five years, a national expert.
- Take an online course (we offer courses at amenuniversity.com).
- Cross-train at work. Learn someone else's job. Perhaps you can even look into switching jobs for several weeks. This benefits the business and employees alike, as both workers will develop new skills and better brain function.
- Break the routines of your life to stimulate new parts of your brain. Do the opposite of what feels natural to activate the other side of your brain and gain access to both hemispheres. Write

or brush your teeth with your nondominant hand, shoot basket-balls with both hands, become a switch hitter when you play baseball, play table tennis or use the computer mouse with your other hand—making your brain feel uncomfortable exercises it.

Mental exercise is as important to your brain as diet and physical exercise.

4.

Combat Stress with Accelerated Mindfulness

We all experience significant stress on a daily basis—whether it is at home, at work, financially, or within the corridors of our minds. It's a war. Unremitting stress has been associated with many problems in the brain, including atrophy of the memory centers (hippocampus) deep within the temporal lobes; a weakening of the immune system, which makes illness more likely; boosting cravings for sugary foods, alcohol, or drugs as a form of self-medication; and an increase in the production of beta amyloid plaque formation, which is associated with accelerated aging, Alzheimer's disease, and other forms of dementia.

Some stresses are unavoidable, such as moves, job changes, relationship separations, raising teenagers, or taking care of elderly parents. Having a regular, disciplined stress management program is a critical piece of the Brain Warrior's Way. It's essential to learn how to cope with stressors, combat the negative effects of stress, and achieve accelerated mindfulness.

Here are five daily habits we find particularly helpful.

SLOW YOUR BREATHING, ESPECIALLY WHEN YOU EXHALE!

Do you know what causes a stress attack? Too much activity in the part of your brain that senses danger. Consciously taking slow, deep breaths (taking twice as long to exhale) helps you regain control. Controlling the breath is part of nearly all meditative practices and is one of the easiest stress management skills to master and practice. Taking five slow, deep breaths several times a day, especially when you feel stressed, will help reset your mind in a positive way. Training "breath" is a key aspect of training soldiers and police officers to decrease the adrenaline response during highly stressful encounters. When adrenaline floods your body as it does in a panic attack, your vision becomes limited, hearing is altered and decision making is affected. If it helps soldiers and police officers who experience some of the most stressful situations imaginable, imagine how much it will help you. Practice this now.

WIN THE WAR BETWEEN YOUR EARS.

> The greatest weapon against stress is our ability to choose one thought over another.
>
> —WILLIAM JAMES

Kill the ANTs. Whenever you feel sad, mad, nervous, or out of control, write down your automatic negative thoughts (ANTs) and ask yourself if they're true and whether they are helping you or hurting you. Thoughts lie; they lie a lot, and it is our unquestioned or uninvestigated thoughts that steal our happiness. Having a thought has nothing to do with whether or not it is true, which is why we call them automatic negative thoughts. They can attack your mind and literally ruin your life. All of us need an internal anteater patrolling the streets of our minds. If you don't question and control your thoughts, the ANTs provide the gasoline for anxiety, depression, and sleep problems and wreak havoc on your relationships. You don't have to believe every stupid thought you have! In many different scientific studies, learning how to kill the ANTs by challenging your negative thoughts has been found to be as effective as prescription medication for anxiety and depression—with no side effects.

■

British author David Gemmel wrote, "Don't speak badly of yourself. For the warrior within hears your words and is lessened by them."

■

Nowhere in school is there formal training on managing your moment-by-moment thoughts, but it is a critical discipline in managing stress. Unexamined negative thinking drives anxiety, depression, and disease, while unexamined positive thinking can also be unhealthy and drive bad decisions and premature death. For example, many people think they can eat low-quality food on a consistent basis and nothing unfortunate will happen to them. Brain Warriors are "accurate, honest thinkers," constantly monitoring what they think and asking themselves if their thoughts are true, helpful, and mission-driven.

People err when they allow their thoughts to become too negative or too positive. It is important to have more balanced thinking. One of our favorite New Testament verses is John 8:32, "Ye shall know the truth, and the truth will set you free." Monitor your moment-by-moment thoughts. Pay attention to what you are thinking and evaluate your thoughts for their helpfulness and truthfulness. Whenever you notice you have an ANT infestation, the best way to rid yourself of the pesky creatures is to write down your thoughts and investigate them. Turn your ANTs into PETs (positive empowering thoughts). The empowering thoughts are honest, true, motivating, and helpful.

For example, if you are in a theater and crave the popcorn that is loaded with genetically modified, pesticide-sprayed corn, poor-quality fat, and a boatload of salt, ask yourself, "Does this fit my goals?" Likely it does not. Of course, you are likely to win the war against the popcorn if you ate nutritious food before going to the theater and have a good blood sugar level.

A common ANT in this situation is, "I can never have any fun when I go out. I feel deprived." Yet, if you eat the food, you are depriving yourself of what you want most, which is health, energy, creativity, a strong memory, and a positive mood.

An overly positive thought in this situation is "I can have a large bag of popcorn. I deserve it after eating well all week." The more bad decisions you make, the harder it will be to make good decisions.

Common ANT Myths

Over the years we have heard many myths about health that people truly believe, such as:

You just need more willpower, which will never work by itself when faced with purposefully addictive foods. It is like telling an alcoholic to stop drinking and just try harder. You need the whole plan.

It's your own fault is one of the most devastating myths. The health of our society is going the wrong way. Your health has been sabotaged at every turn. Until now, no one has taught you to become a Brain Warrior.

You can't lose weight, which is often funny because many overweight people have lost hundreds of pounds, but cannot sustain it because they are on a diet—not changing their lifestyles permanently.

It's all genetic, which is a lie. Only 20 to 30 percent of health problems are related to genetic inheritance. An article in *Nature* reported that even cancer was due to environmental or behavioral factors 70 to 90 percent of the time.[116] There is so much you can do to become and stay healthy and prevent future problems once you understand what to do.

Don't let the ANTs and myths steal your happiness and rob your health. Be careful how you talk to yourself. Your unconscious mind and the child within are listening. We often ask our clients if they would speak to their children the same way they speak to themselves. Many times they say no. It is a good barometer of what is appropriate. With practice, you'll have a choice about which thoughts you allow yourself to think.

HEART RATE VARIABILITY TRAINING

There is a powerful connection between your brain and heart. Research has shown that when you experience positive emotions such as kindness, gratitude, joy, empathy, and compassion, you produce synchronized rhythms in your brain (coherence). When you experience negative or toxic emotions such as anger, frustrations or hopelessness, you produce erratic rhythms (lack of coherence). Positive or negative emotions can also impact your heart rate variability (HRV), which is the beat-to-beat variation in heart rhythm. This in turn can affect your ability to adapt to physical, emotional, and environmental stresses.

HRV training is a simple way to lower stress and accelerate mindfulness. Most people think that a healthy heart rhythm is perfectly regular, but in a healthy heart it is not. Even under normal, healthy conditions, our heart rhythm fluctuates. High HRV has been associated with heart and brain health, while low HRV has been associated with illness.

HRV issues can become apparent when mothers deliver babies. Obstetricians typically use scalp monitors to monitor the baby's HRV before delivery. In a healthy baby, the heart rate varies significantly. If the baby's heart rate becomes too steady, the baby is considered to be in trouble. Lower HRV is a sign of distress, whether we are about to be born or are adults. HRV has been found to predict survival after a heart attack. Over a half dozen well-designed studies have shown that reduced HRV predicts sudden death in patients who have had a heart attack.[117] Studies also suggest that lower HRV may predict the risk of death even among individuals free of heart disease.[118] Knowing what you do now about the relationship between our brains and our physical health, it might not surprise you to learn that studies also show a relationship between high levels of anxiety and heart disease.

Many other studies have suggested a link between negative emotions (such as anxiety and hostility) and reduced HRV.[119] One research group reported an association between anxiety and reduced HRV in 581 men, while another group observed lower HRV in individuals who were "highly anxious."

The exciting news is that you can easily train your HRV. We often recommend HRV trainers, such as those found at HeartMath (heartmath.com). They have an Inner Balance iOS app, a stand-alone device (emWave2), and a computer program (emWave Pro) that both kids and adults love. Many professional athletes are able to avoid injury and increase performance by using HRV training.

PRAYER, MEDITATION, SELF-HYPNOSIS, AND GUIDED IMAGERY

Decades of research have shown that prayer, meditation, visualization, and self-hypnosis can calm stress; improve focus, mood, and memory; and enhance overall brain function. Taking 5 to 10 minutes twice a day to focus on your breathing, gratitude, loving-kindness, a beautiful scene in nature, or scriptures is simple, yet can have a powerful effect on your life.

Self-Hypnosis: Here is a simple form of hypnosis we do with our patients and clients and one you can do on yourself.

- Sit in a chair or lie on your back with your hands at your side.
- Pick a spot on a wall or the ceiling that is a little bit above your eye level. Stare at the spot. As you do, count slowly to twenty. Notice that in a short while your eyelids begin to feel heavy. Let your eyes close. In fact, even if they don't feel as if they want to close, slowly close them anyway as you get to twenty.
- Next, take a deep breath—as deep as you can—and very slowly exhale. Repeat the deep breath and exhale slowly three times. With each breath in, feel your chest and belly rise and imagine breathing in peace and calmness. With each breath out, feel your chest and belly relax and blow out all the tension, all the things getting in the way of your relaxation. By this time, you'll notice a calm come over you.
- Next, tightly squeeze the muscles in your eyelids. Close your eyes as tightly as you can. Then slowly let the muscles in your eyelids relax. Notice how much more they have relaxed. Then imagine that relaxation spreading from the muscles in your eyelids to the muscles in your face—down your neck into your shoulders and arms—into your chest and throughout the rest of your body. The muscles will take the relaxation cue from your eyelids and relax progressively all the way down to the bottom of your feet.
- After your whole body feels relaxed, imagine yourself at the top of an escalator. Step on the escalator and ride down, slowly counting backward from twenty. By the time you reach the bottom, you're likely to feel very relaxed.
- Then add relaxation imagery. In your mind choose a haven that promotes deep relaxation, such as a beach, park, mountain lake, or forest. Your haven can be a real or imagined place, as long as it makes you feel safe and relaxed. Imagine it with all five senses. See, hear, feel, smell, and taste what is there. For example, at a beach, see the water, hear the sounds of the waves and the birds calling, feel the warm sand between your toes or the breeze on your skin, smell the fresh ocean air, and sense the faint taste of salt on your tongue.
- After a few minutes of imagining your haven, get back on the escalator and count to ten as you ride up to being fully awake.

To make these steps easy to remember, think of the following words:

FOCUS (focus on the spot)
BREATHE (slow, deep breaths)
RELAX (progressive muscle relaxation)
DOWN (ride down the escalator)
IMAGERY (experience your haven with all of your senses)
UP (to be fully awake)

The first several times you do this, allow yourself plenty of time. Some people become so relaxed that they fall asleep for several minutes. If that happens, don't worry. It's actually a good sign—you're really relaxed!

If you want to have Daniel as a personal guide in this process, you can join our Brain Fit Life community (mybrainfitlife.com) and listen to our hypnosis audios.

Research has shown that self-hypnosis can increase heart rate variability; lower blood pressure; increase circulation; aid digestion; strengthen the immune system; improve cognition; and diminish feelings of anxiety, depression, and irritability.[120]

Loving-Kindness Meditation: New research has also shown many positive benefits of a special form of meditation called loving-kindness meditation (LKM), which focuses on developing feelings of goodwill, kindness, and warmth toward others. LKM has been shown in scientific studies to increase positive emotions and decrease negative ones,[121] decrease pain[122] and migraine headaches,[123] decrease symptoms of post-traumatic stress disorder[124] and social prejudice,[125] increase gray matter in the emotional processing areas of the brain,[126] and increase social connectedness.[127]

To practice LKM, sit in a comfortable and relaxed manner with your eyes closed. Take two or three deep breaths—taking twice as long to exhale. Let go of any worries or concerns and feel your breath moving through the area around your heart. LKM is practiced first toward ourselves, because if we have difficulty loving ourselves, it is harder to be loving and compassionate toward others. As you sit, quietly or silently repeat the following or similar phrases:

May I be safe and secure.
May I be healthy and strong.
May I be happy and purposeful.
May I be at peace.

While you repeat these phrases, allow yourself to really feel the intentions they express. LKM focuses on connecting to the positive intentions. As you repeat these phrases allow the feelings to grow deeper.

After a few repetitions, direct the phrases to someone you feel thankful for or someone who has helped you:

> *May you be safe and secure.*
> *May you be healthy and strong.*
> *May you be happy and purposeful.*
> *May you be at peace.*

Then, visualize someone you feel neutral about—people you neither like nor dislike—and repeat the phrases.

Then, visualize someone you don't like or with whom you are having a hard time. Kids who are being teased or bullied at school often feel quite empowered when they send love to the people making them miserable.

Finally, direct the phrases toward everyone universally: *May all beings be safe and secure.*

You can do this for 10 minutes or 30 minutes. It is up to you.

Guided Imagery: This is a mind-body technique that uses positive sensory and mental images to enhance various aspects of a person's life. It is commonly used as an adjunct tool in psychotherapy as well as in sports psychology to help athletes achieve their goals. Tana used guided imagery as part of her training for her second black belt. Tana knew she would need to prepare on four fronts:

> *Biological:* Sleep, hydration, supplements, strength, and superior health
> *Psychological:* Meditation, visualization, eliminating the ANTs
> *Social:* Relying on her tribe for support, practice, and honesty about needs for improvement
> *Spiritual:* Spending regular time in prayer and focused on purpose

But in this case, none would be more important than the *psychological* front. She already knew the curriculum and was well trained. She was healthy and strong. Her community was behind her. However, at the age of forty-six, having to take high-dose thyroid medicine for chemother-

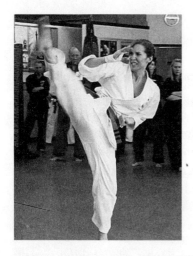

apy for her recurrent thyroid cancer that always kept her heart rate elevated, Tana knew that she would need to win this fight mentally above all things. She would need to go into the test well rested and not overtrained, so as the test date came closer, she relied more and more on guided imagery and less on physical training.

Many, if not most, Olympic athletes incorporate imagery into their training routine. Coaches who train high-level athletes know that they can help their athletes perform better by teaching their brains to focus with perfect execution on various scenarios over and over. The technique is referred to as imagery instead of visualization because it helps athletes use all of the senses and imagine in as much detail as possible their upcoming event.

Nicole Detling, a sports psychologist with the U.S. Olympic Team, explains, "The more an athlete can imagine the entire package, the better it's going to be. . . . In images, it's absolutely crucial that you don't fail. . . . You are training those muscles, and if you are training those muscles to fail, that is not really where you want to be. So one of the things I'll do is if they fail in an image, we stop, rewind and we replay again and again and again."

Dan Coyle, author of *The Talent Code*, explains that imagery can be used for nearly any new skill. He describes it this way: "This process of learning skills changes the hardware in which knowledge is stored in our brains—the more we learn, the more it changes. It is also like downloading new software, meaning the inner circuitry of your PC (brain) becomes upgraded from Pentium 1 to Pentium 4. Experts possess the most up-to-date software . . . you can only get this upgrade by thousands of hours of practice."

Imagery can give you a shortcut by helping reinforce the groups of brain cells responsible for new skills simply by just thinking about those skills. Done in the right way it can be a close second to actual physical practice, as shown by an experiment in which three groups were given a new task to perform: One with no practice, one with mental practice only, and a third with physical practice only. The no-practice group improved very slightly. The physical-practice group improved the most, but the mental-practice group improved nearly as much over ten days. This shows how massively important mental practice (imagery) is.

There are many different uses for imagery, including the following:

Past performance accomplishments: Imagine or recall yourself doing your previous best performances—for example, the best bits from your last competition or while training. This is especially good before competition with music or if suffering a confidence crisis. Remind yourself how good you can really be if you apply yourself.

What-ifs: Use imagery to mentally practice all possible scenarios before your next event or competition—the "what-ifs?" For example, what happens if I have transportation or relationship issues? You can also practice using all the mental toughness exercises, such as positive self-talk, to overcome any problems. In this example, research alternative transportation or how to deal with relationship troubles. This also can be used for what might happen in the competition (for example, how to deal with a hostile crowd).

Dealing with pressure: During the competition, use mental exercises like self-talk to practice how to react to situations that may cause a breakdown in discipline—that is, how you will react to showboating, bad refereeing, concentration lapses, or making mistakes.

Mental rehearsal: Practice the technical/tactical areas you need to identify to be successful.

Downloading information: Rehearse the technical/tactical information you have taken on during the day from a training session and try to add it into your current knowledge. This way it will boost the groups of brain cells and the cell-covering myelin responsible for those skills.

Mistake correction—the three F's: Try to remember where you went wrong in previous competition or training or when making mistakes during competition if you have time and focus. How can you avoid those mistakes again? Remember, don't dwell on the mistakes; just concentrate on putting them right and imagining yourself doing the correct technique.

To be used during mental imagery after mistakes to prevent you from thinking negatively.

1. Fix it: What did you do wrong and what can you do next time to reduce the chances of making the same mistake? This helps you rehearse the correct way to do things and should be used in future imagery instead of the mistake.
2. Forget about it: There's no point in dwelling on mistakes; just learn from them and move on. This way you can avoid being negative about your performance and treat mistakes as they should be treated—as a part of the positive learning experience.
3. Focus: Get back on track; refocus your mind on the task at hand (self-talk might be used here). Put it behind you, but also get your mind back on the job at hand. *Concentrate!*

MAKE A BRAIN-ENHANCEMENT PLAYLIST

Used properly, music is medicine. Music can soothe, inspire, and help you focus. In Barry Goldstein's powerful book *The Secret Language of the Heart*,[128] he reviews the neuroscience properties of music. "Music stimulates emotional circuits in the brain."[129]

"Releases oxytocin, the cuddle hormone, which can enhance bonding, trust, and relationships."[130] . . .

"Listening to music can create peak emotions, which increase the amount of dopamine, a specific neurotransmitter that is produced in the brain and helps control the brain's reward and pleasure centers."[131]

"Music was used to assist patients with severe brain injuries in recalling personal memories. Music helped patients to reconnect to memories they previously could not access."

Music pieces specifically composed by Goldstein to enhance creativity, mood, memory, gratitude, energy, focus, motivation and inspiration can be found at mybrainfitlife.com. Treat your brain and listen often.

Other music to consider for your playlist are the following:

BRAIN WARRIOR MOTIVATION

Song: Artist

"Warriors": Imagine Dragons

"Brave": Moriah Peters

"Battle Cry": Skillet

"Get Over It": The Eagles

"Fighter": Christina Aguilera

"Chariots of Fire": Vangelis

GRATITUDE

"Thank You for This Day": Karen Drucker

"Thank You": Dido

LOVE

"Love Can Build a Bridge": The Judds

"All of Me": John Legend

JOY

"Joy to the World": Three Dog Night

HAPPY

"Happy": Pharrell Williams

"Om Mantra": Deva Premal and Miten

RELAXATION

"Wisdom of the Heart": Monroe Institute

"La Isla Bonita": Madonna

"Dolphin Dreams": Jonathan Goldman

"Awakening": Jonathan Goldman

"Weightless": Marconi Union

"Wisdom of the Heart": Barry Goldstein

PEACEFULNESS

"Watermark": Enya

SLEEP

"Deep Theta 2.0 (Part 1)": Steven Halpern

"Delta Sleep System (Part 1)": Jeffrey Thompson

"Adagio for Sleep": Liquid Mind

"Just the Way You Are": Bruno Mars
Sonata for Two Pianos in D Major, K. 448:[132] Mozart
"Silk Road": Kitaro

5.

Make Sleep a Priority

As discussed in Part 2, healthy sleep is absolutely essential to a brain healthy life and Brain Warriors protect their sleep as if it were one of the most important things they ever do—because it is. Sleep rejuvenates all the cells in your body, gives brain cells a chance to repair themselves, helps wash away toxins that build up during the day, and activates neuronal connections that might otherwise deteriorate due to inactivity. Sleep is also necessary if you want to have glowing skin, high energy, a sunny mood, excellent health, and stable weight.

Unfortunately, as many as 70 million Americans have trouble sleeping and it is progressively getting worse with the proliferation of gadgets and bad habits. In 1900, Americans averaged nine hours of sleep. According to a recent Sleep in America Poll, Americans now average only six hours and forty minutes. Even more disturbing, the percentage of people getting less than six hours of sleep has risen from 12 percent in 1998 to 20 percent in 2009, while the percentage of Americans getting a good eight hours a night has decreased from 35 percent in 1998 to 28 percent in 2009.

Sleep problems come in many varieties. Do you have trouble falling asleep? Do you go to sleep easily but wake up repeatedly throughout the night? Do you find it hard to drag yourself out of bed in the morning? Do you or your significant other snore? All of these problems can lead to decreased brain function and a weaker body. Getting less than seven hours of sleep a night has been associated with lower overall brain activity, which can affect your weight, your skin, your mood, your health, your athletic performance, and most important, your decision making. Insomnia causes lower activity in the prefrontal cortex and temporal lobes, affecting attention, judgment, impulse control, memory, and learning. Considering all of this, it is no surprise that sleep-deprived individuals struggle to maintain a healthy mood, memory, or body.

In a survey from the Better Sleep Council, 44 percent of workers admitted that when they are sleep deprived, they are more likely to be in an unpleasant or unfriendly mood. Studies show that decreased motivation due to poor sleep makes you more likely to skip family events, work functions, and other recreational activities. Social connections help keep the brain young, so missing out on get-togethers and events due to fatigue can dampen your mood and prematurely age your brain. Plus when you are sleep deprived, you are less inclined to exercise or get intimate with your significant other, which deprives your brain and body of feel-good chemicals that boost your mood. If you want to improve your mood, improve your sleeping habits. When you don't get enough sleep, you are inclined to gulp more caffeine, smoke more, exercise less, eat more junk food, and drink more alcohol.[133] Studies show that sleep-deprived adolescents are also more likely to drink alcohol, smoke marijuana, and use other drugs than those who get enough sleep. Sleep deprivation is also associated with obesity,[134] type 2 diabetes, depression, anxiety, ADHD, and psychosis.

Getting the sleep you need requires three strategies:

1. Get sleep envy (you have to see it as critically important).
2. Avoid sleep robbers.
3. Engage in sleep enhancers.

AVOID SLEEP ROBBERS

In our hectic, 24/7 society, we could just as easily ask, What doesn't cause sleep deprivation? There is seemingly an endless number of reasons why millions of us are missing out on a good night's sleep. Here are some of the most common factors:

- A warm room
- Light in the bedroom
- Noise
- Gadgets by the bed
- Going to bed worried or angry
- Medications: Many disturb sleep, including asthma medications, antihistamines, cough medicines, anticonvulsants, and stimulants (such as Adderall or Concerta for ADHD).

- Caffeine: Too much coffee, tea, chocolate, or even some herbal preparations—especially when consumed later in the day or at night—can disrupt sleep.
- Alcohol, nicotine, and marijuana: Although these compounds initially induce sleepiness for some people, they have the reverse effect as they wear off, which is why you may wake up several hours after you go to sleep.
- Restless legs syndrome: A nighttime jerking or pedaling motion of the legs that drives a person's bed partner crazy (as well as the person who has it).
- Women's issues: Pregnancy, PMS, menopause, and perimenopause cause fluctuations in hormone levels that can disrupt the sleep cycle.
- Snoring: It can wake you or your sleep mate or everyone in the house if it is really loud.
- Sleep apnea: With this condition, you stop breathing for short periods of time throughout the night, which robs you of restful sleep and leaves you feeling sluggish, inattentive, and forgetful throughout the day.
- Shift work: Nurses, firefighters, security personnel, customer service representatives, truck drivers, airline pilots, and many others toil by night and sleep by day. Or, at least, they try to sleep. Shift workers are especially vulnerable to irregular sleep patterns, which leads to excessive sleepiness, reduced productivity, increased irritability, and mood problems.
- Stressful events: The death of a loved one, divorce, a major deadline at work, or an upcoming test can cause temporary sleep loss.
- Jet lag: Travel across time zones wreaks havoc with sleep cycles.
- Several health conditions can also interfere with sleep, such as
  - Thyroid conditions
  - Congestive heart failure
  - Chronic pain conditions
  - Untreated or undertreated psychiatric conditions (obsessive-compulsive disorder, depression or anxiety)
- Alzheimer's disease: Dementia patients may "sundown" or rev up at night and wander
- Chronic gastrointestinal problems, such as reflux.

■ Men's issues: Benign prostatic hypertrophy causes many trips to the bathroom at night, which interrupts slumber.

ENGAGE IN SLEEP ENHANCERS

Here are twenty-one ways to make it easier to drift off to dreamland and get a good night's sleep. Remember that we are all unique individuals and what works for one person may not work for another. Keep trying new techniques until you find something that works.

■ A cooler room.
■ A completely dark bedroom.
■ Make the room noise free or wear earplugs.
■ Turn off the gadgets by the bed or at least turn off the sound.
■ Try to solve emotional problems before going to sleep with a positive text, e-mail, or intention to deal with the issue tomorrow. If you forgive the other person first, you may just end the argument.
■ Maintain a regular sleep schedule: Go to bed at the same time each night and wake up at the same time each day, including on weekends. Get up at the same time each day regardless of sleep duration the previous night.
■ Create a soothing nighttime routine: A warm bath or shower, meditation, or massage can help you relax and encourages sleep.
■ Read yourself to sleep: If you are reading, make sure it isn't an action-packed thriller or a horror story—they aren't likely to help you drift off to sleep.
■ If you are having trouble sleeping, don't take naps! This is one of the biggest mistakes you can make if you have insomnia. Taking naps when you feel sleepy during the day compounds the nighttime sleep cycle disruption.
■ Sound therapy can induce a very peaceful mood and lull you to sleep. Consider soothing nature sounds, wind chimes, a fan, or soft music. Studies have shown that slower classical music, or any music that has a slow rhythm of sixty to eighty beats per minute, can help with sleep.[135] You can find sleep-enhancing music by Grammy Award–winning producer Barry Goldstein on Brain Fit Life (mybrainfitlife.com).

- Drink a mixture of warm unsweetened almond milk, a teaspoon of vanilla (the real stuff, not imitation), and a few drops of stevia. This may increase serotonin in your brain and help you sleep.
- Don't eat for at least 2 to 3 hours before going to bed.
- Regular exercise is very beneficial for insomnia, but don't do it within 4 hours of the time you hit the sack. Vigorous exercise late in the evening may energize you and keep you awake.
- Wear socks to bed. Researchers have found that warm hands and feet were the best predictors of rapid sleep onset.
- Don't drink any caffeinated beverages in the afternoon or evening.
- If you wake up in the middle of the night, refrain from looking at the clock. Checking the time can make you feel anxious, which aggravates the problem.
- Use the bed and bedroom for only sleep or sexual activity. Sexual activity releases many natural hormones, releases muscle tension, and boosts a sense of well-being. Adults with healthy sex lives tend to sleep better. When you are unable to fall asleep or return to sleep easily, get up and go to another room.
- Hypnosis or meditation can help. We have audio downloads on mybrainfitlife.com that could be helpful.
- Use the scent of lavender to enhance sleep. It has been shown to decrease anxiety, improve mood, and enhance sleep.[136]
- Natural supplements, such as melatonin, 5-HTP (especially for worriers), magnesium, and GABA, may be helpful.
- If you have to resort to medication, stay away from the benzodiazepines and traditional sleep medications because of their negative effects on the brain. Daniel uses trazodone, gabapentin, and amitriptyline with his patients.

6.

Protect Your Decision-Making Skills

The best way to reduce stress is to stop screwing up.

—ROY BAUMEISTER, PhD

For most people, their health and overall success in life are the sum of all the decisions they've ever made. When someone is not healthy or struggles to be successful, it is likely he made thousands of bad decisions. When someone is the opposite, it is likely the quality of her decisions was much better. You don't have to get all your decisions right, but the more you get right, the better you are likely to look, feel, and act. In fact, if you improve self-control in one area of your life it improves it in other areas. For example, if you start walking every day, you are also likely to start eating better.

Consistently making great decisions is not hard if you put your brain in the position to help you make them. Here are the most important strategies for boosting the quality of your decisions:

- Start with clear focus. Know your goals (One Page Miracle) and look at them every day.
- Make decisions about your brain health ahead of time. It is good to have a few simple rules, such as eating no bread or drinking alcohol at restaurants before meals, as they both lower prefrontal cortex function and have a negative impact on decisions.
- *Do not allow yourself to get hungry!* Hunger is the enemy of good decisions. Eat breakfast with high-quality protein to balance your blood sugar levels daily. Low blood sugar is associated with lower overall blood flow to the brain. A high-carbohydrate breakfast can sabotage your day and your decisions. Willpower is tied into your body's energy supply. Continue to eat small amounts throughout the day to maintain healthy blood sugar levels. In one of the most fascinating studies, researchers measured the blood sugar levels of 107 married couples right before bedtime. Then they gave each spouse voodoo dolls and asked them to express their feelings about their partners by putting the pins in the dolls. The people who had the lowest blood sugar scores stuck more than twice the number of pins in their dolls.[137] Protect your blood sugar levels—your marriage and maybe even your life could depend on it. One of Daniel's patients used to make headline news by getting herself arrested on a regular basis. When we tested her blood sugar it was dangerously low, which was likely associated with irritability and poor decisions. One of his strongest recommendations was that she should keep food with her at all times to keep her blood sugar stable.

- Eliminate sugar and artificial sweeteners. These often trigger cravings and poor decisions.
- Get at least 7 hours of sleep at night. Less than that is associated with lower blood flow to the brain and more bad decisions. We both travel a lot, but do not schedule flights before 10:00 A.M. Otherwise our decision-making ability on tour will likely suffer.
- Don't put yourself in vulnerable situations. Think ahead. If you know you are going to a party that is likely to serve unhealthful food, eat before you go so you won't feel hungry and lose control. We often bring food with us to gatherings, just to have something in case of emergency low blood sugar or cravings. The Greek myth of Odysseus is a great example of not putting yourself in vulnerable situations: He wanted to hear the Sirens' song even though he knew that doing so would render him incapable of rational thought. On advice, he put wax in his men's ears so that they could not hear and had them tie him to the mast so that he could not jump into the sea. Upon hearing the Sirens' song, Odysseus was driven temporarily insane and struggled with all of his might to break free so that he might join the Sirens, which would have meant his death. It would have been better—and easier—for him if he chose another way home.
- Keep a journal to help keep you focused, accountable, and on track. It can also help you double your weight loss, according to a 2008 study from Kaiser Permanente's Center for Health Research. Many of our patients and clients have used journaling successfully to make massive gains in their health. Once they start a healthy habit and journal about it for 2 weeks or more they do not want to break the streak and stick with it. In Part 7, you'll find the 14-Day Brain Warrior's Way Journal to use as an example. It is essential to know the simple habits you are supposed to strengthen each day and then write them down, reinforcing them until they become second nature. It takes only a few months, but if you journal, you can strengthen the brain circuits that will serve your health for the rest of your life. For example, if you notice you are struggling with cravings or having a hard time making good decisions, a journal will tell you where you might have gone wrong, such as if your sleep is off, you forgot to eat breakfast, you went too long between meals,

you were under excessive stress, or spent time with unhealthy people. If you can discover the pattern of your vulnerable times, you can then develop strategies to overcome them. In your journal, focus your mind on your biggest temptations, obstacles, and excuses and write them down. Record your temptations and look for patterns, such as time of day, sleep, stress level and so forth. Learn from your mistakes; they are your best teachers, especially if you are curious, rather than just harshly judging yourself. Know your triggers for both good decisions and poor decisions. Be aware of the land mines in your life.

WHAT WE CAN LEARN FROM TWO-YEAR-OLDS WITH RAISINS AND FOUR-YEAR-OLDS WITH MARSHMALLOWS

A simple test on twenty-month-old toddlers using raisins can predict how the child will perform in school at the age of eight.[138] Using raisins under an opaque plastic cup, the test was based on how long the kids could wait before they picked up the raisins. After several training sessions, they were asked to wait until they were told 60 seconds were up before they could eat the raisins. The children who were born prematurely, and thus likely to have frontal lobe trouble, were more likely to impulsively take the raisins before time was up. The study found that those who had trouble inhibiting their behavior were more likely to struggle in school up to seven years later. Likely they struggled for the rest of their lives, unless someone helped remediate their brains or spent time teaching them to delay gratification. Willpower is a muscle that must be practiced to stay strong. In our experience, you can improve it even if you were born prematurely or had a brain injury.

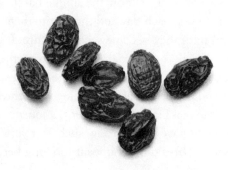

This is not a new idea. In the 1960s, psychologist Walter Mischel invited preschoolers, one at a time, into his lab, where there was a marshmallow on a table. He told each child that they had two options. They could either eat the marshmallow right away or they could wait for several minutes and then get two marshmallows. Some of the children couldn't wait and gobbled up the marshmallow. Others used an array of tactics to keep from eating the treat to get two, such as clapping their hands or turning their chair to face away from the marshmallow. You can find several reenactments of this landmark experiment by searching for "marshmallow test" on YouTube. Mischel then followed these youngsters for fourteen years and found that those who were able to delay gratification fared much better in life than those who ate the marshmallow right away. The "waiters" had higher self-esteem, were better at coping with stress and frustration, performed better academically (scoring an average of 210 points higher on their SATs), and were more socially adept.

In a follow-up study, Mischel did the experiment with adults modeling delayed gratification. The grown-ups used a variety of tactics to avoid eating the single marshmallow while the youngsters watched. Then, when it was their turn to reign in their impulses, children who previously had eaten the lone marshmallow used the techniques they had just witnessed and successfully managed to wait it out and get two marshmallows. In a later follow-up, these children performed at levels similar to those who had the natural ability to delay gratification. Children and adults can learn techniques and strategies to make good decisions. If kids can do it, so can you! Learn the art of distraction when you are tempted—sing a song, take a brief walk, or meditate on your goals for a few moments.

CAN YOU WAIT FOR MARSHMALLOWS?

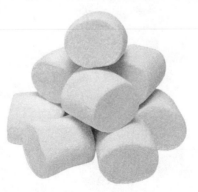

7.

Be Curious, Not Furious. Become Masterful at Learning from Your Mistakes

You will become clever through your mistakes.

—GERMAN PROVERB

Be curious, not furious about relapses or setbacks. You have to fall to learn how to walk. The same thing is true for learning to be a lifelong Brain Warrior. In order to change, you have to be armed and prepared for the inevitable roadblocks and setbacks that will come your way. It is critical to identify your most vulnerable moments and have a plan to overcome them. Change is a process! If you pay attention, the difficult times can be more instructive and helpful in the long run than the good times. Take bad days and turn them into great data.

We often go to the whiteboards in our offices and draw the following diagram.

When people come to see us they usually are not doing very well. Over time, if they work with the plan we develop, they get better. But no one gets better in a straight line. They get better, then there is a setback,

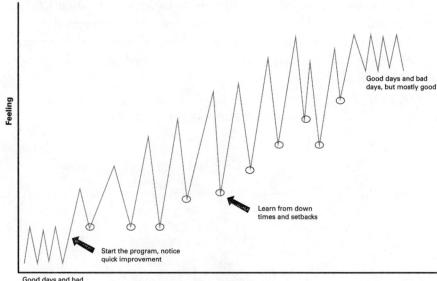

BE CURIOUS, NOT FURIOUS

Good days and bad days, but mostly good

Learn from down times and setbacks

Start the program, notice quick improvement

Good days and bad days, but mostly bad

Feeling

Time

then they get better still, then there may be another setback, then they continue to improve. Over time, they reach a new steady state where they are consistently better. The setbacks are critically important if you pay attention to them. They can be your best teacher.

Do you learn from your failures or ignore them? New brain imaging research suggests that when some people fail, their *motivation* centers become more active, making it more likely they will be able to learn from their experience. They are driven to overcome problems. When others fail, the brain's *pain* centers become more active—it literally hurts—making it more likely they will do whatever they can to avoid thinking about the episode, meaning they are more likely to avoid the lessons and thus to repeat the same mistakes. Learn from your mistakes and use them as stepping-stones to success.

Many of our clients and patients have found it helpful to create simple rules for vulnerable times, such as:

1. Eat healthful foods before bad ones, like Brain Warrior Nancy.
2. Split and share large entrées.
3. Eat salad and veggies first.
4. Eat something before you go to the ball game or concert to avoid being tempted by the caramel apples.
5. Use smaller plates; you put less on them and thus eat less.
6. You can cheat on your diet, but only after calling a friend, which introduces distraction, delay, and social support.
7. Have a plan for when you experience cravings or feel out of control—take a walk, drink a glass of water (you may be thirsty, but misperceive it as hunger), play Tetris until the impulse goes away (it actually decreases cravings).[139]

If you are truly going to change, you have to change what brings you pleasure! Learn how to find what you love about great low-calorie, highly nutritious food. Learn to find what you love about exercise. One of our friends hated running, but loved playing table tennis. Willpower is a skill, and if people can distract themselves for just a minute, their temptations often go away.

Connect to who you are becoming . . . think like a healthy person. How would a healthy person order this meal? The simple act of identifying yourself as a "Brain Warrior," someone who is a healthy role model to others, can be enough to change the way you see yourself and the way you behave.

BRAIN WARRIOR JACKIE

By being curious and learning from her struggles, Jackie was able to get her bulimia under control. She started to do much better within just a few weeks. We were so pleased with her progress until one day she came in, looking defeated. She'd had a relapse. Rather than be disappointed in her we were curious. "What can we learn? We want to know all about what happened."

It turned out Jackie was following the Brain Warrior plan to the letter. Then late one Friday evening she agreed to meet friends who had come from out of town. She was excited to see them. One of her friends ordered margaritas for the whole table, just as they did in college. Rather than make one decision to not let her friend order the alcohol for her, her anxiety caused her to sit quietly and just go with the group. "I won't drink it," she thought to herself. But because it was on the table she began to fantasize about the salt, sugar, and bittersweet taste. The more she tried to use her willpower, the less it seemed to work for her. Pretty soon she had drunk the whole glass and started to feel remorseful. Then the nachos came and again she promised herself she wouldn't eat any, but the alcohol lowered the activity in her prefrontal cortex, the judgment and impulse control center of her brain, and she ate more than she wanted. Feeling disgusting and terribly bloated she went to the restroom and made herself throw up.

As we investigated the events of the day, we found several important learning opportunities and helped her to create strategies for the future.

If Jackie goes to meet friends later in the evening, she must eat ahead of time to make sure she has a good blood sugar level, so she can make good decisions. Going to a place where there is any alcohol means Jackie needs to have a brain that is fully armed with great nutrition ahead of time. She had skipped eating earlier in the day before she went out with her friends.

We practiced dealing with friends who are food pushers. Never let someone else order drinks for you. If Jackie would have ordered for herself, she would have ordered sparkling water and lime. When her friend ordered the alcohol, she allowed her social anxiety to cause her to remain silent, which set her up for the alcohol that lowered her judgment centers and made her more vulnerable to the nachos.

We taught Jackie the acronym we teach all patients and clients to prevent relapse: HALT, which stands for not letting yourself get too:

Hungry—it lowers your blood sugar and overall blood flow to the brain thus making you more prone to making bad decisions.

Angry or anxious—negative thought patterns have also been shown to decrease overall brain function and decrease good decision-making skills.

Lonely—social isolation diminishes feedback from others and increases depression and the potential for self-medication. Jackie wanted to fit into the group.

Tired—a lack of sleep is associated with lower blood flow to the prefrontal cortex, which decreases the quality of your decisions. Jackie slept poorly the night before because she stayed up late to work on a project.

Being curious about the times you struggle is essential to learning from them.

ELEPHANT AND THE RIDER WARS

We like the metaphor of the elephant and the rider to help us visualize two forces in the brain that are often in opposition. The prefrontal cortex (PFC) is the rider: It is the thoughtful part of your brain that attempts to direct your life. The PFC is also called the executive part of the brain, like the CEO at work, and is involved with planning, forethought, judgment, and impulse control. The limbic or emotional brain is the elephant. It is the powerful, emotional part of you that drives your impulses and desires. As long as the elephant wants to go where the rider directs him, things work fine. But when the elephant "truly, deeply, madly" wants to go somewhere that the rider prefers him not to go, who is going to win that tug of war? Most bets

(CONTINUED)

are on the elephant. Cravings (elephant) are often controlled by the PFC (rider) when things are going well, but if the elephant is spooked or becomes nervous or afraid, it can stampede out of control.

How do we then integrate the rider and the elephant, so that our PFC and limbic brains, our goals and our desires, our thoughts and behaviors, are more in sync? We do it through continual training, in the same way animal trainers train powerful elephants. You tame the inner elephant with clear goals, ANT-free thinking, healthy sleep, blood sugar stabilization, and by always protecting your PFC (which is easily damaged by brain injuries).

Think of this scenario: Your inner elephant really wants a large pastry and nudges you toward the sugar high. But, as a Brain Warrior, you have trained your brain to pause and think about the consequences of the pastry: the fatigue, mental fog, diabetes, and excess weight. You want a more positive outcome, so you make a different choice, such as slicing an apple and adding some almond butter for a healthy snack, which satisfies your cravings and calms the elephant down.

God gave you a big brain for a reason. The rider has a proportionally bigger brain, in order to make good decisions.

Prefrontal Cortex:
Decision-making part of
the brain (judgment and
impulse control)

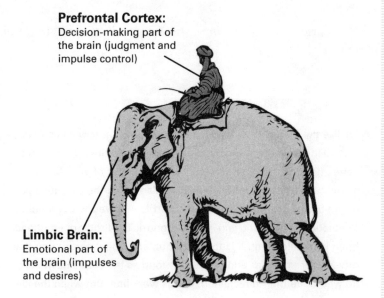

Limbic Brain:
Emotional part of
the brain (impulses
and desires)

Brain Warrior Training Takeaways

1. Start each day with intention, gratitude, and appreciation.
2. Engage in smart exercise.
3. Flex the muscles between your ears.
4. Combat stress with accelerated mindfulness.
   - Slow your breathing, especially when you exhale!
   - Kill the ANTs.
   - Practice heart rate variability (HRV) training.
   - Practice prayer, meditation, and self-hypnosis (loving-kindness meditation).
   - Make a brain enhancement music playlist.
5. Make sleep a priority.
6. Protect your decision-making skills.
   - Have a clear focus.
   - Plan.
   - Maintain healthy blood sugar, not too high or too low.
   - Eliminate sugar and artificial sweeteners.
   - Sleep.
   - Eliminate vulnerable situations.
   - Keep a journal.
7. Be curious, not furious. Become masterful at learning from your mistakes.

PART 5

Essence of a Brain Warrior

Transform Your Pain into Purpose

Fate whispers to the warrior, "You cannot withstand the storm," and the warrior whispers back, "I am the storm!"

—AUTHOR UNKNOWN

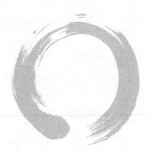

A CRY THAT CHANGES THE WORLD

In fiction, without Darth Vader there is no Luke Skywalker. In real life, without apartheid most of us would never have known the name Nelson Mandela. Without a foe, there is no warrior journey. Too many people—including us—bitch, moan, and complain about the hardships in our lives, feeling they may be unfair. Yet, it is through our trials that our gifts can emerge, and it is by overcoming temptation and troubles that we are made stronger and more valuable to the planet. Your gifts reflect your "essence," which refers to the passion deep within that stirs your soul. It can be described as your spirit or the "spirit of a warrior" and is often born out of frustration and pain.

In Part 1, we explained the importance of knowing your *why*, your motivation for being healthy. Your essence is different from motivation, though they are often linked. Your why could be as simple as "I'm sick of feeling sick" or "I want to live a long, healthy life." That is great motivation, but it isn't essence. Your essence is connected to something bigger and more important than just yourself.

When a warrior cries it is from deep within his or her core being; it is cultivated from his or her essence, not from superficial wounds. It's a cry from emotional pain, injustice, and witnessing the suffering of others. Warriors are passionate about what really matters and they don't hide it. A warrior's cry changes families, communities, nations, and even the world.

BRAIN WARRIOR RABBI G

Our friend Rabbi Elimelech Goldberg (affectionately called Rabbi G) has a warrior cry that can be heard around the globe, resonating his desire to ease the pain and suffering of hurting children.

Rabbi G held his tiny, limp, and lifeless daughter in his arms as she passed away at age two from leukemia. It was a brutal and gruesome battle. Though his heart was split open through her suffering, he took comfort in the wisdom she spoke to quell his anguish, words well beyond her earthly knowledge. As her skin sloughed off her body a bit more each day from the treatments she endured, she would politely tell the nurses, "No medicine today please." She would lie on her father's chest in his futile attempt to comfort her. Instead she comforted her father, telling him, "It's okay, Abba. I love you." In her final hours she smiled and looked at her father with a determined look. When asked where she wanted to go, this little soul pointed up to heaven.

Rabbi G's life was shattered. He couldn't possibly make sense of this horrible event with his earthly wisdom. But his faith in God gave him strength to survive a tragedy no parent should have to endure. He believed in a purpose much greater than himself and greater than the cancer that took his very young daughter away from their family to be with angels in heaven. Without that faith his life would have no meaning. He believed wholeheartedly that God had an important job for him. God had a plan for his life and it wasn't for him to argue or question. God's plan soon became clear.

In 1999, Rabbi G founded a nonprofit organization called Kids Kicking Cancer. Through a coincidental encounter (if you believe in coincidence), Rabbi G became the director of a summer camp for children with cancer. One day, he walked into the infirmary, which was like a little hospital in the woods, and witnessed a five-year-old child screaming terribly while being held down by two nurses. A third nurse was attempting to plunge a large needle into this little boy's chest for his chemotherapy. When the rabbi entered, he was so overcome with the little boy's cries that he yelled out "Wait!" and they did. Even the child stopped screaming. "I'm a black belt," the rabbi told the child. "May I teach you some karate?" The little boy almost jumped off the table. "In karate they teach us that pain is a message you don't have to listen to." Together they engaged in a simple tai chi breathing technique. Twenty minutes later, the nurse took out the needle. The boy looked at her and asked, "Did you do it yet?" That's when Kids Kicking Cancer was born.

Through Kids Kicking Cancer, Rabbi G and his skilled staff of psychologically minded martial artists teach hospitalized children with debilitating pain from cancer and other diseases to think and act like martial artists. He teaches them meditative breathing techniques to help

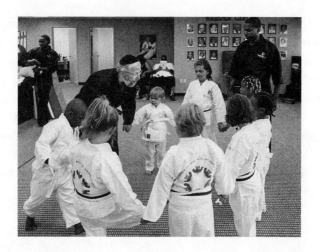

them "breathe in light and breathe out pain." He puts tiny gis (martial arts uniforms) on these pint-size warriors, often bald from chemotherapy and has them do empowering moves to emphasize what they can do instead of focusing on what they can't. The results have been astounding! Instead of screaming when the health-care professionals come in to administer treatments, many of these courageous little fighters begin to refuse to be held down, opting for their new martial arts skill as a coping mechanism instead. Sometimes they even refuse pain medication. Their new declaration is often, "I'm a martial artist! You don't have to hold me down. I won't cry! I'm powerful!"

Rabbi G now travels the globe, coaching qualified black belts to become instructors for his cause. He's been featured with the children on *Good Morning America* and the *Early Show* as well as in *People* magazine. In 2014, Rabbi G was featured as a Top Ten CNN Hero. His warrior cry is changing the world and making it a better place. Rabbi G is someone we look up to because he transformed his personal pain into passion to empower others.

KIAI: THE WARRIOR CRY

Chi or ki, common terms in martial arts, are defined as "the harmonious joining of body, mind, and breath." Chi means spirit. Utilizing the loud kiai, the practitioner learns to focus on chi to obtain maximum power.

(CONTINUED)

Kiai, the shout warriors make in fighting, literally translates to "expression of spirit." It reminds us to breathe. It expresses our spirits. It has a psychological effect on us and the attacker, boosting our confidence, while intimidating the attacker. It gives us energy. And, when you breathe deeply it settles down the stress hormones that are released with the adrenaline response. As discussed in Part 4, at Amen Clinics, we use deep-breathing exercises to induce relaxation and self-control for patients, so they can defeat their enemies—the attacks of anxiety and fear. In this way, breathing exercises, like the kiai, help people realign the mind, body, and spirit.

WHAT WOULD YOU SUFFER FOR?

Brain Warriors are passionate. This passion often stems from having experienced or witnessed deep suffering or pain in the past. In fact, the Latin root for the word *passion* is *pati*, meaning to "suffer" or "endure." You love someone so much you would suffer for them, such as the passion of Christ. It's not mandatory that Brain Warriors have had pain in the past that has touched their souls, but in our experience, it is commonly found in the most passionate Brain Warriors. The pain of a Brain Warrior isn't always directly personal pain, as in Tana's fight with cancer. As with Rabbi G, the passion may come from witnessing the suffering of others, especially people we love.

Where do you hurt? How have you suffered in the past? Who have you seen suffer? How can you turn your pain into a passionate cry that can transform your life, your community, or even the world? You may not see yourself as that important; most people with an important mission didn't see themselves that way in the beginning. Usually it starts with a desire to stop your personal suffering, or the suffering of someone you love.

DISCOVER YOUR PURPOSE

Your essence and your spirituality are intertwined. They cannot be separated. One of our favorite definitions of spirituality comes from Christina Puchalski, founder of the George Washington Institute for Spirituality & Health, who wrote, "Spirituality is that which gives meaning to one's life and draws one to transcend oneself." While this often includes religion, it is a much broader idea. It's about how you express your spirit in the world and connect to a larger purpose. Prayer, meditation, giving back, and having a relationship with God or a "higher power" are the expressions of your spirituality. The simple act of practicing these strategies on a daily basis can give you clarity, decrease anxiety, and help you see a greater purpose. In multiple studies, having a deep sense of meaning and purpose is associated with a longer life.[140] In one study of over 9,000 people with an average age of sixty-five, researchers found that those with the greatest sense of purpose were 30 percent less likely to die during the eight-and-a-half-year follow-up period than those with the least sense of purpose.[141]

One of our favorite questions to help people focus their energy outward (away from self) to discover their purpose is, Why is the world a better place because you breathe? If you don't know the answer to this question, it is worthwhile to take some time to think about it. What skills do you have that could be helpful to someone today? What can you do to make the world a better place?

In our clinics we see many patients who feel disconnected. They lack a sense of meaning and purpose. They lack a relationship with God or something bigger than themselves. Regardless of religion, denomination, or even personal belief in God, a lack of meaning and purpose in life can lead people to feel alone, depressed, and insignificant. It doesn't have to be that way.

STEPS TO FINDING YOUR ESSENCE

Clear your mind and meditate on the following questions or journal your thoughts and responses to them.

1. Get in touch with past or present pain and injustice in your life. Where in your body do you feel it? Where does it hurt?

2. Think about what you are truly passionate about. What connection might there be to your suffering?

3. What are you willing to suffer for? Write down the things you believe in so strongly that you would fight for them without concern about criticism or ostracism.

(CONTINUED)

4. What are your thoughts and feelings about passion? Journaling often helps people become aware of the behaviors that drive them.
5. Meditate or pray daily with intention about that for which you are passionate or in your quest to discover what it is you are most passionate about.
6. Ask yourself, Why is the world a better place because I breathe? If you aren't sure, start journaling your personal skills, interests, and passions and ask yourself what small step you could take today—and every day—to make a difference, to create happiness and healing in the world.
7. Find someone with passion whom you respect and ask him to mentor you.
8. Mentor someone. The most effective way to create lasting change and increase your passion for something you love is to mentor someone else and watch her grow. As she flourishes, so will you.

There is one significant difference that distinguishes Brain Warriors from others who have suffered. Brain Warriors get up after they've been knocked down. Like sheepdogs, they fight and survive where others may fail. Many people who suffer great pain and injustice become devastated. Many don't recover or learn to cope effectively. Many use food, drugs, alcohol, or sex as their form of self-medication or become a victim to their tragedy, allowing pain to be the excuse they use to hurt themselves. Brain Warriors can also struggle, but they keep trying and they rely on their community when they feel weak. They know scars form a stronger barrier that protects them from future pain. *Brain Warriors transform their pain into the passion that fuels their mission to make the world a better place!*

Brain Warriors know their purpose and are less affected by the words *I can't*. In fact, pain sometimes fuels their passion. Our friend Jacob is a wonderful example of a Brain Warrior who doesn't let the words *I can't* dictate his destiny, despite his pain.

BRAIN WARRIOR JACOB:
CHALLENGED, BUT NOT DISABLED

With passion, intention, and a plan, amazing things can happen. As Tana was gasping for air at the completion of her grueling three-hour black belt test in Kenpo in May 2015, one of the master instructors, Ken Kellogg, approached her to ask if she would mind taking the time to meet a fellow martial artist who was a fan of hers and Daniel's. Master Ken explained that Jacob had shown up that day to watch her test and hoped to meet her. Honored, Tana followed but was initially surprised to meet Jacob. Sitting in his wheelchair, Jacob gave Tana one of the biggest, most infectious, slightly crooked smiles she had ever seen. Jacob has lived with cerebral palsy since birth. Tana knew immediately that there was something special about Jacob. He virtually glows with happiness and enthusiasm. But she was a bit thrown off by the "fellow martial artist" comment, considering it took *everything* in her power not to pass out during most of her lessons, and she's pretty fit. She couldn't imagine how Jacob, with cerebral palsy, could pull it off. She knows the community he trains with. They don't give pity or honorary belts. But one thing both Tana and Daniel know is that people with passion can accomplish far beyond what their challenges or situations dictate.

Jacob always inspires us with his drive and positive attitude, but never more so than when he received his brown belt in Kenpo. He's been training intensely for years, using what he has as weapons. He elevates his wheelchair, swings, throws back knuckles and even grabs his opponent in choke holds. Jacob is always pushed to his limits, and he loves it! The secret to Jacob's success is never letting his limitations be an excuse to give up.

When Tana congratulated him, he was quick to give all of the glory first to God, then to his instructors and fellow students who consistently help him. We love what he said: "I'm thankful for the instructors and friends who don't treat me like I'm disabled." Jacob purposely does not spend time with people who handicap him, and neither should you. As a result, he lives an extraordinary life for which he feels blessed and thankful to God every day. *That is essence!*

Having Jacob as a friend can make it more challenging at times for us to not become frustrated when people tell us, "I *can't* do it because it's hard" or "I'm too old" or "I'm too tired" or almost any other excuse. When you say "I can't," you disempower yourself. Your subconscious doesn't have a sense of humor. It just does what you tell it. To break this pattern, we will often show Jacob's picture and say, "I didn't quite get that. Could you remind me why you can't do it? Be honest. If you're just not willing or don't want to do it, just say so, but please don't say you *can't*!"

Brain Warriors are not fearless, but they are *fierce!* When you become a Brain Warrior, courage takes over where fear used to be crippling. Courage isn't the absence of fear; it's the willingness to do something even when you're absolutely terrified. Mothers and fathers are usually attuned to this feeling. In spite of fear, and often *because* of it, parents willingly die to protect their children. They use fear as a warning sign that says, "Something is dangerous, pay attention. Be ready to protect those you love." That's the intensity, passion, and courage we want you to channel into being a Brain Warrior. This is about protecting yourself and the people you love from what may be threatening their safety.

Parents of special needs children are often the most fiercely protective. They have to be. They live in a daily war zone. They are constantly fighting a medical system that does not always work smoothly for more or better care, more rights, and protection of their children. They are on the clock 24/7, watching for seizures, vomiting, abnormal breathing, diarrhea, temperature spikes, and subtle changes in cognition. They watch for bed sores and infections. And sadly, because many of these children can't communicate effectively, they must always be on high alert to protect their children from predators who prey on the weak and helpless. There is literally no rest for many of these mothers and fathers.

We know this from experience. Our granddaughter, Emmy, who suffered with seizures and still struggles with language and developmental

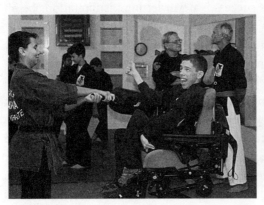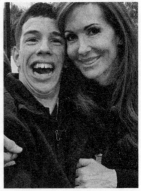

delays, has parents who will do anything to help her. The constant need to watch their precious children wears many of these mothers and fathers out. They get depressed, tired, overwhelmed, and often their marriages suffer, because of the intense focus on their children. We marvel at their sheepdog dedication, but also know they will protect their children more effectively if they take care of themselves, their marriages, and their brains. As you always hear when on a plane, "When the oxygen masks come down, put yours on first so you can be there to take care of those who need you."

BRAIN WARRIOR LISA

Lisa Ackerman is the founder of Talk About Curing Autism (TACA), which came out of the need to help her son and all of the families who struggle with autism. It was born out of pain but now serves tens of thousands of families worldwide. In Lisa's own words:

> In September 1999, the word "autism" rang through my ears like a cannon shot across the bow. My husband and I knew something was not going well with our son Jeff, but we would have never guessed it was autism. Following that fateful visit with the neurologist, we visited many other professionals including medical doctors, speech pathologists, audiologists, and behaviorists. The list seemed endless. The common message we were given: *Autism has no hope, no cure.* In fact, the first three medical doctors recommended that my family find "institutional placement" for Jeff who was the ripe old age of 2½ years at the time. Refusing to give up on our son, my husband and I spent hundreds of hours talking to any and all parents of children diagnosed with autism, reading dozens of recommended books, watching countless hours of educational videos, and of course, surfing the Internet constantly. We were determined that our beloved son would grow far beyond his label and that he would have a future that was wonderful and amazing despite his autism diagnosis. Early on, the most important step for us was to GET BUSY. It was up to us, HIS PARENTS, to make a difference for his future.

The early days of our son's diagnosis were frustrating. Those countless hours spent researching, reading, talking—wasn't there a better way? Wasn't there SOMEONE who had already done the same research before, who could have brought us up-to-speed much sooner for us to help our son faster? Fast-forward to November 2000 when our daughter Lauren (at the advanced age of 16) recommended that we start a parent support group. Both my husband and I felt we were not qualified but we definitely wanted the company of other families going through the same struggles, for social gatherings and to share information, especially new research and treatment options as they became available. We also hoped to build a community where parents would be inspired by each other's steadfast hopes for their children's futures and who would be passionate about autism education for themselves and other similarly struggling families, as well as raising awareness in the general public.

TACA began with a small handful of families in a living room in 2000. In 2016, we serve almost 50,000 families around the United States. From a grassroots beginning in Southern California, TACA expanded nationwide and now has a physical presence via our Chapters in 24 states and a virtual presence in the rest of the nation.

Where is my son Jeff now? He is a teenager at a typical high school, learning the same curriculum as his peers with a great grade point average. He attends school dances and events. He has applied for college. He talks, makes jokes, gives out hugs, runs on the high school cross-country team, socializes with friends, and is an active member of the society with a bright future. He also happens to be the sweetest, kindest person I know and is practically always smiling. That is a far cry from his early diagnosis and the initial prognosis for his future.

TACA's goal is to provide education, support, and information to parents to help their children diagnosed with autism be the very best they can be, with the hope of recovery.

Today, there are many, many treatment options that help alleviate many of the symptoms suffered by our children diagnosed with autism. Let us share our collective, hard-won knowledge and experience with your family so your child's

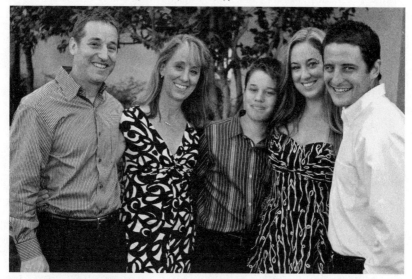

treatment can begin right away. Ask about the autism journey because we are families with autism who have already "been there and done that" with many of our children. Some of us are still working hard every day with our children for whom we never give up hope. We are **Families with Autism Helping Families with Autism.**

The autism journey is not an easy one. It's a marathon, not a sprint; so take each minute, hour, or day, one at a time. It will be difficult, but it will also be incredibly rewarding, because it will change your life, your family's life, and most importantly, the lives of your children with autism so we all enjoy a brighter future.

Born out of pain, Lisa is passionate to help families with autism stay together. Helping other families is in her essence, her soul. Visit tacanow. org to learn more about TACA.

Like Rabbi G and Lisa, the mission or purpose of Brain Warriors is personal. It matters. Their passion and desire to help others gives them the ability to deal with any criticism that comes their way. They realize that the purpose for which they were chosen is much bigger than they are as individuals. Even if you were once debilitated by the opinions of others or by the need to be popular or "perfect," after you get in touch with your true purpose, you will no longer be driven by what others think. Perfectionism, by the way, is a disease that many of us seem to be born with and it is a roadblock to our success. It's incredibly liberating when you realize that you weren't put on this planet to see how many popularity votes you can acquire—you're not getting a "most popular" trophy at the end of your life. You were put here to make the biggest difference you can, with the gifts you were given.

BRAIN WARRIOR COLONEL (RETIRED) JILL CHAMBERS

Colonel Jill Chambers was working inside the Pentagon on 9/11, just two corridors away from where the plane crashed through the building. "They were all my friends—all people that I had grown with over the last twenty-five years. I stopped going to funerals after my eleventh one because I just couldn't do it anymore," Jill told us in an interview.

For many years, she didn't talk about the burning aircraft that chased her in nightmares or mention that she had insomnia and couldn't get more than 3 or 4 hours of sleep at night. Like so many others with post-traumatic stress disorder, she had brushed the issues off as "a normal part of life now."

Fast-forward to 2007 when suicides among service members were skyrocketing. Admiral Mike Mullen, the chairman of the Joint Chiefs of Staff, asked Jill to serve as the first special assistant for Returning Warrior Issues. Jill was solely tasked with pinpointing the *ground truth* about transitional challenges facing wounded service members and developing dynamic, real-time strategies and recommendations. Admiral Mullen was committed to ensuring that under his watch, no fallen comrade would be left behind. He empowered Jill to work with that end in mind.

In 2008, General George Casey Jr. publicly honored Jill for her work and launched the Comprehensive Soldier and Family Fitness Program, focused on the army's five dimensions of strength: social, emotional, family, spiritual, and physical. After decades of denial, the U.S. Armed Forces finally started talking about and addressing the psychological well-being of service members and their families.

Jill was thrilled with her accomplishments and made the decision to retire in April 2009. Once retired, she realized that she too had post-trau-

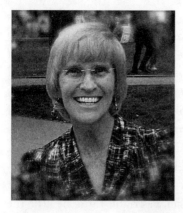

matic stress disorder from the events on 9/11 and committed three solid months to focusing exclusively on her mental and physical health. A doctor friend introduced her to neurofeedback and guided imagery, which completely changed her life. By the end of August, Jill was sleeping better and hasn't had a nightmare since. Her newfound passion for integrative healing therapies led her to Daniel's book *Change Your Brain, Change Your Body*. She developed brain envy and committed herself to practicing the Brain Warrior's Way. A true warrior, Jill stopped eating wheat and sugar, began monitoring her important health numbers, and joined Brain Fit Life, our online brain-enhancement program. Jill reported on her success using the program:

> I build focus with the brain games and then I am able to consciously bring that focus into other areas of my life. I also watch the video lessons a lot. I can take 7 minutes out of my night or my morning to build my confidence and resilience by learning something new. I love it. If I would have had this tool [Brain Fit Life] 10 years ago while working in the Pentagon, I would have been unstoppable!

Not only has Jill been successful in improving her own health; she is now paying it forward through her own nonprofit, This Able Vet (ThisAbleVet.com). Her program is free to veterans who are ready to take responsibility for their own health. She empowers and equips veterans with the same brain-focused tools and resources that Jill uses in her own life. Jill turned her pain into passion. She found her essence.

TANA'S STORY: PAIN SHARED IS PAIN DIVIDED

In my early twenties, after dealing with a lifetime of bad health, I finally gave up and succumbed to the dark cloud of depression that had been threatening for years. I was convinced God had given up on me and saw no purpose to my life. It was actually me who had given up, not God, but I couldn't see past my own pain to see that there was a special plan for my life. How could I know I would feel my best and be able to transform my pain into a passion for helping others decades later in my *forties?* When I met Daniel, he began encouraging me to share my story with others, to teach them how to heal the way I had. But this meant venturing into terrifying territory . . . *vulnerability! There was no way I was about to tear down the carefully built walls that had taken me decades to build.* The truth of my story was simply too painful. I was sure that if people knew how chaotic and unglamorous my life had been, how many mistakes I had made, how ugly it all was, they would never accept me, let alone listen to me. I was sure of one thing: People wanted a perfect message from a perfect messenger, even if it was a facade.

Over time I slowly realized that Daniel was right. Little by little the walls came down and real healing began to take place. Joy replaced fear and anger. By tapping into the past pain I can relate to depressed patients who lack a sense of purpose. *Pain shared is pain divided. Joy shared is joy multiplied! Pain divided is joy multiplied.*

My new prayer was that God would use me as a messenger, and He does. This is a gift. It is my purpose, passion, and essence. To disregard it would be to reject a gift from God.

What is your essence, your passion, your purpose for breathing? If you do not know, now would be a good time to ask yourself that question, again and again.

Brain Warrior Essence Takeaways

Find your essence by turning your pain into purpose.

Who or what would you suffer for?

Being disabled is a state of mind.

Never let the opinions of others dictate your life's strategy.

Ask yourself, Why is the world a better place because I breathe?

PART 6

Responsibilities of a Brain Warrior

Building and Protecting Your Brain Warrior Tribe, Now and into the Future

Example isn't another way to teach—it is the only way to teach.

—ALBERT EINSTEIN

The fastest way to get healthy is to find the healthiest person you can stand and spend as much time as possible around him or her.

—DANIEL AND TANA

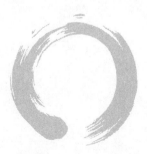

BRAIN WARRIORS ARE SERIOUS, RELENTLESS, AND RESPONSIBLE

Your life is not just about you; it is about generations of you, literally. A new field of genetics, called epigenetics, has exploded onto the scientific scene in the last twenty years. *Epigenetic* means "above or on top of the gene." It refers to the recent discovery that your habits, emotions, and environment can turn on or off certain genes, making illness more or less likely in you as well as in your children, grandchildren, and even great-grandchildren. Your habits, feelings, and environment impact your biology so deeply it causes changes in the genes that are transmitted to the next several generations. It is these epigenetic "marks" or "etches" that tell your genes to switch on or off or to express themselves more loudly or softly. It is through epigenetics that immediate environmental factors like diet, stress, toxins, and prenatal nutrition can affect the activity of the genes that are passed to your offspring and beyond. This reminds us of the harsh wisdom of Exodus 34:7. "He punishes the children and their children for the sin of the parents to the third and fourth generation."

A 2006 study showed that boys who started smoking cigarettes before puberty (say at age eleven or twelve) increased the risk of obesity in their children.[142] A dumb decision at age eleven can impact generations to come. And obesity[143] is just the beginning. Some researchers believe that epigenetics holds the key to understanding certain cancers,[144] forms of dementia,[145] schizophrenia,[146] autism,[147] diabetes,[148] and even panic and fear.

Are you afraid of something and have absolutely no idea why? Brian Dias and Kerry Ressler from Emory University[149] did an experiment where they made mice afraid of the scent of cherry blossoms by mildly shocking them whenever the scent was in the air. This is called classical conditioning, akin to what Ivan Pavlov did with his dogs in the 1920s. Dias and Ressler's amazing discovery was that the first- and second-generation offspring were also afraid of the scent of cherry blossoms; the fear was transmitted down through generations through the etchings the shocks made in their genes, even though the younger mice were never exposed to the shocks. The implications of this research are far-reaching: Emotions like fear, anxiety, and perhaps even hatred and prejudice may have generational origins. Prior generational stress has also been associated with depression, antisocial behaviors, and memory impairment. Fortunately, stress in your ancestors can go both ways. For example, another study suggested prior generational stress can help animals learn to better cope with adversity.[150]

Epigenetic changes often serve to prepare children and grandchildren for an environment that is similar to their parents' to help them survive. But when the environment is toxic, as it is today in a world that's gone crazy with unhealthy choices and pollution, we have the potential to literally damage our future selves.

◼

You speak your love to your children and grandchildren by your actions today. Brain Warriors are responsible to their future loved ones.

◼

THE RIGHT SOCIAL CONNECTIONS MAKE YOU SMARTER; THE WRONG ONES HURT YOU

People have banded together to form tribes from the beginning of time. The reason is simple—survival. Modern lone warriors don't fare much better today than they did in prehistoric times. Humans are hardwired to be social creatures and need bonding. According to biologist E. O. Wilson, all people (no exception) need a group to which they belong, show loyalty and jockey for power, *and even to demonize the enemy.*

The same power that makes a tribe victorious is the power that makes it vulnerable—and sometimes even dangerous. That's why you have to choose your tribe carefully. But it is the quality of the social connections that really matter. It's critical for a tribe to have a clear code of ethics and values and not get distracted by herd mentality. Remember, sheep aren't very smart and will follow other sheep right off the cliff!

BENEFITS OF BELONGING TO A TRIBE

- Support
- Membership
- Safety
- Belonging
- Influence
- Bonding and connection
- Loyalty
- Accurate feedback from people you trust
- Different views on solving problems
- Motivation to stay healthy

New results from the Framingham Heart Study showed that social connections among the elderly positively correlated with the level of a protein called brain-derived neurotrophic factor (BDNF), which is involved with memory, learning, and a reduced risk of dementia and stroke.[151] More social connections were associated with higher levels of BDNF, while fewer connections were associated with less. Increased BDNF levels have been implicated in a range of behaviors that protect the brain, including eating a lower-calorie diet and exercise. Increases in BDNF also encourage the growth of new neurons and the formation of connections between neurons that improve communication.

VULNERABILITIES AND DANGERS OF A TRIBE

- Swayed by others' unhealthful habits
- Can override individual thinking
- Can create herd mentality
- Can create discrimination against other tribes
- Decreases empathy for other tribes
- Us versus them mind-set
- Can stifle creativity by demanding tradition

The people in your tribe are contagious. Whom you spend time with matters. The people close to you can affect how long you live and how happy you are, so it is important to be selective because people affect your brain, mood, and physical health. A number of studies report that if you spend time with people who are unhealthy, their habits tend to rub off on you. A study published in the *New England Journal of Medicine* found that one of the strongest associations in the spread of illness is the people with whom you spend the most time. The research was conducted on over 12,000 people who participated in a multigenerational heart study collected from 1971 to 2003. The study showed that if a person had a friend who became obese, they had a 57 percent higher chance of becoming obese themselves. This number went up to 171 percent if both friends identified the other as a strong friend. Friendship was apparently the strongest correlation; it didn't matter how far away the friends lived, as geographic distance proved a negligible factor. Sibling influence was also ranked high, with an increased 40 percent chance of becoming obese if another sibling was obese. And, as we discussed earlier in this book, obesity is associated with many health problems, including depression and dementia.

The study highlights the "social network effect" on health issues and makes an important point: Our health is heavily influenced by many factors, not the least of which are the role models around us. The powerful influence of friendship works both ways.

■

Researchers also found that when health-conscious friends improve their health, their friends' health improves as well.

■

By becoming a Brain Warrior you can influence your whole network of friends and family to live healthier and happier lives. If you lead the way to better health in your circle of friends, your friends and their loved ones will also benefit. The author of the study said, "People are connected, and so their health is connected." People can connect to improve their lives through walking groups, healthy cooking groups, meditation groups, new learning groups, and so on. When you spend time with people who are focused on their health, you are much more likely to do the same.

Engaging others to be healthy is a win-win. It's helping you, and it is helping them. Just as when we become emotionally healthy as individuals, our relationships improve, so it is with our physical health. If we get physically healthy, it tends to be contagious and our relationships improve in terms of more activity, eating better, feeling well, and looking younger. What a gift to receive, give, and share!

BRAIN WARRIOR JUDY

About a year after we started the Daniel Plan with Pastor Warren and Mark Hyman, we were leaving a service at Saddleback Church one Sunday when Judy approached us and said she had lost 45 pounds.

"Congratulations," Tana said to her, but the woman said that was not the point of the story.

"What do you mean?" Daniel asked.

"When I first started, I realized we were doing all the wrong things at home. Fast food, lots of treats and sugar, and supersizing everything because we thought it was a good value. My husband was 300 pounds and all five of our children were overweight. I was horrified when I learned about epigenetics. Our poor decisions were condemning our children and grandchildren to ill health."

"Using new information to get healthy is the sign of intelligent life," Tana interjected.

"But my husband wouldn't get on board. He said it was just a fad and all the health-scare stuff was overblown. I knew he was wrong, but remembered what Dr. Amen taught us. Don't nag others if they won't join you. Lead by example."

"Nice," Daniel said.

"Well, I did tell him I would be happy long after he was dead, but it was only once."

We laughed.

"But as I got really healthy and lost 45 pounds, my husband started to pay attention. He wanted the energy I had and has now lost 75 pounds and is in great shape. All of our kids are on board with the new way of living too and they have more energy and are even doing better in school. We all support each other. We are not leaving a legacy of illness, but one of health."

What about you?

Think about the people with whom you spend time. Your life just might depend on it! Do these five things to create a healthier tribe today:

1. Have a clear vision for your life and your tribe—focus on it daily. For example, "I am a living example of health and fitness and belong to a tribe that believes the same."
2. Be the change you want to see and don't shy away from or be afraid of criticism. Eventually, people come around.
3. Protect the relationship, so that at some point the people who are slow to get on board are still connected to you. Don't be a jerk about it. Be firm and kind.
4. Keep the sheepdog mind-set. Sheepdogs don't ever do anything that will hurt the flock.
5. If your current tribe is entrenched in a hostile or negative mind-set, make sure to build new tribe members who believe and act as you want to.

We created the Brain Warrior's Way to help you build a tribe of like-minded people to get and keep healthy. Ultimately we want you to get healthy and then help or inspire another tribe member to get healthy too. There are too many sheep in the world. We need more sheepdogs, more leaders, more people focused on making positive changes in themselves, their tribes, and the world. To do that effectively you need to be surrounded by other like-minded people—other Brain Warriors!

You can do remarkable things on your own, but by creating your own tribe, you can be an even greater agent for change when your efforts are magnified by the power of community. Linda Wagener, a leadership consultant, says, "If I can only give people one piece of advice about how to make a change, I'll recommend that they surround themselves with people who embody that change."[152] There are a number of specific reasons for why being part of a community that supports change is so helpful, she explains. First, it provides a mirror to us, so we see ourselves more truly without underestimating or overestimating our strengths and weaknesses. We can use that information to make our actions more effective. Working with others also gives us the encouragement to go beyond what we think we can do. This is important when we're nervous about trying something new. Community also provides accountability to follow through on what we promise. We're more likely to visit the gym every day or take that brisk walk if we have a friend who is waiting for us to show up. Furthermore, a health-conscious tribe gives us the support we need when we get discouraged and want to quit.

The power of community also has the opportunity to influence peers in a positive way. In her book *Join the Club: How Peer Pressure Can Transform the World*, Tina Rosenberg talks about the "social cure."[153] She explains that when people try to bring about change, they usually do it by sharing information in an attempt to convince others. But the social cure takes a more direct approach. It changes behavior by helping people get what they care about most, which is the respect of their peers. Rosenberg believes that social pressure through a peer group—what she means by a club—is the best way to influence behavior. The peer group (tribe) is so strong and persuasive it can cause people to adopt a new identity as a member of the club. And they emulate the behavior of other club members: "I can be like my friend whose life has changed."

Possibly the most famous and successful of these clubs is Alcoholics Anonymous. Put someone with others who have the same goal and together they form an entity that pressures each individual to meet the group goal. Researchers give us some insight into why participating in a group can be so effective. First, being part of a tribe helps relieve chronic stress, thus removing a key factor in obesity, memory problems, cardiovascular and digestive issues, insulin resistance, and a weakened immune system. On the positive side, being in a supportive group elevates stress-reducing hormones like oxytocin (the chemical associated with bonding). That's why getting together with your friends for a chat when there is a lot of bonding going on can lead to a euphoric kind of peace, as long as it doesn't involve wine, cookies, or cheesecake.

Rosenberg believes that much of the dissatisfaction people have in life is due to feeling isolated. People are seeking community and connection. The social cure may involve a sacrifice of time for meetings and a loss of privacy, but it solves important personal problems and adds meaning to people's lives. Getting others to join you in your endeavors is a great way to improve your chances of success.

As much as good company keeps you on track, bad company, as we have said, can derail you, so again, be aware of the kind of company you keep! The power of social influence cuts both ways, and if you spend time with people who are unhappy and negative or who engage in unhealthful habits, they can bring you down instead of raising you up. Clearly, we influence each other for good or for bad. Be mindful of the influences around you. But also take this as a powerful motivator to be a good role model and a positive influence on the people with whom you interact. We know that when health-conscious friends improve their own health, their friends' health also improves. You can be the one who encourages others to do better by doing better yourself.

And the more you help others, the more you will help yourself. We like to think of it this way: *You have to give it away to keep it.* We saw a great example of this one evening at an event in our home. Tana runs a group through Amen Clinics to help women lose weight and get healthy. To celebrate the last class of the session, Tana held a party for the group members. During it, we got into a conversation with one of the women who told us she had taken the class to learn how to deal with fibromyalgia and brain fog. Within two weeks of starting the program, the fibromyalgia symptoms were gone and her mind was much clearer. She had also dropped 11 pounds, which had been her goal. She said that she felt our program had changed her life. We congratulated her on her progress and told her that to keep improving she had to give the program away by teaching others what she had learned. She replied that she had already begun. Her husband and children had started to eat better, and she was sharing information about healthy food instead of cookies with her coworkers. She had learned for herself that when you share your knowledge with others, you more firmly embed that wisdom into your daily life.

This is how you can be the agent for change: Reach out to others so you can get healthy together helps both of you. And there are many benefits to your health, your well-being, the way you look and feel, and the quality of your relationships. It's a win-win for everyone—*and it all starts with you.*

TANA: HURT PEOPLE HURT PEOPLE

I'm going to be very vulnerable and admit something pretty ugly about myself. When I began volunteering to help the Salvation Army's largest chemical addiction recovery program to implement our brain health program, I was suddenly filled with horrible judgmental thoughts about the addicts in the program. It's clear that clean eating helps people with addictions make better decisions so I wanted to help. But how could I help people who brought up feelings of fear and loathing inside of me? You see, most of the participants (beneficiaries) are court ordered to be in the program, and many go there after having served time in jail for some pretty serious criminal offenses.

Growing up, I directly experienced the consequences that drugs can have on people. I hated drugs and had no tolerance for anyone who did them! When I told Daniel I didn't think I could follow through with helping at the Salvation Army, that God had picked the wrong person this time, he smiled in that very annoying way husbands (and psychiatrists) often do. He said, "God picked the perfect person."

He was right. Working with that population gave me new empathy for their backgrounds, which were not much different from my own. And I realized that for every person I could help, **there would be one less scared child in the world.**

It truly is in the giving that we receive. Sometimes, helping others is the best way to heal our pain from the past. The revelation I found staring me in the face was, *Hurt people hurt people.* While I don't make excuses for criminal and hurtful behavior, reaching past our own pain and understanding the root cause of such behavior is the first step in creating long-term solutions and healing. In other words, relax your guard and drop your shield long enough to see the world through another's eyes. You don't have to agree, but you can't effect lasting change from across the canyon.

ONCE YOU KNOW THIS INFORMATION, IT'S YOUR RESPONSIBILITY TO ACT ON IT!

For you to have a positive effect on others you need to do everything you can to make sure that your own brain is healthy and working in top condition. Brain Warrior responsibilities require you to:

- Keep your brain and the brains of those you love safe by avoiding toxic foods, chemicals, and illicit drugs and by staying away from dangerous activities that could traumatize your brain or theirs.
- Stabilize your weight at a healthy level and gently encourage others to do the same.
- Get exercise that keeps your blood flowing, especially to your brain, and preferably do it in a group.
- Get sufficient sleep every night and resolve problems like sleep apnea.
- Keep your brain flexible and active by exercising it and learning new information.
- Resolve issues like ADHD, depression, anxiety, and stress by getting appropriate help.
- Surround yourself with a network of supportive people who will encourage your efforts and help you stay on your healthy program.
- Take action to be the change you want to see with fun, creative ways of engaging members of your tribe. For example:
  - Encourage family and friends to join you for exercise with group walks, hikes, and bike rides
  - Teach your children and friends the brain healthy recipes you're learning
  - Start family game night or invite friends to trivia or other memory games
  - Make doctor appointments for your family to address any health issues that may be harming brain function if left untreated

These things won't happen on their own, and no one will do them for you. You must be conscientious of your own health. This is not only for your own good but for the good of everyone you influence.

And there's only one time when you can make the necessary changes to boost the power of your brain and improve your health, and that time is right now. Putting it off until tomorrow usually means putting it off indefinitely. How long have you been intending to start living differently? Hasn't it been long enough?

BRAIN WARRIOR ALICIA

I am so excited to report that I have lost over seventy pounds! I am living proof that a little exercise can go a long way. I have eaten my way through many of life's challenges, justifying my poor choices by calling them "treats." Then I woke up one day and realized I was going from one treat moment to the next, and it was ruining my body. But what really made me feel sad and guilty was that I was passing my terrible habits on to my children. They were beginning to show the effects of my unhealthy lifestyle. That's when I knew I needed to make changes and became a Brain Warrior. Not only did I find it easy to implement but now my husband and children are following the plan and exercising regularly too. My entire family is healthier and happier as a result! *I have had a very long-term, committed relationship with sugar, but I am happy to say we have finally broken up. Now the biggest treat I can give myself and my family is to be healthy.*

BRAIN WARRIOR LONI

We met Loni at a three-day event we taught together in 2014. During a question-and-answer period with the audience, Loni stood up in front of hundreds of people and told us she was really struggling. In 2013, she discovered her husband, Eric, had hung himself in their home, and she was doing everything she could not to kill herself too. She felt suicidal nearly every day now, but she had four children to look after and couldn't imagine abandoning them. Her mind was racing, she couldn't sleep, and she constantly felt overwhelmed, depressed, and hopeless.

Loni was obese as a child and was teased mercilessly by her siblings and adoptive father. By the time she was a teen she was engaging in self-mutilating behavior because she hated herself. Now at forty, she was diagnosed as having bipolar disorder and PTSD. By the time we saw her, Loni had tried sixteen different medications without success.

When she came to Amen Clinics it was the first time anyone had looked at her brain. The scan helped her feel validated. Her brain was extremely overactive. She kept telling her doctors that she could not turn off her thoughts. Now she could clearly see the evidence of what she was experiencing inside. By using the tools we have outlined in this book, Loni was able to stabilize her moods. She said recently, "I don't think I would have been here today had I not had the opportunity to work with the staff at Amen Clinics."

She had experienced more pain in her childhood and adult life than most could ever imagine. She has carried a tremendous amount of shame, guilt, and a sense of never being good enough throughout her life. We cannot possibly recap all of her journey, but did want to share some of the exciting things that have been happening for Loni over the last two years as she fought to become a Brain Warrior.

For over a year she has worked as a therapist for handicapped children and is extremely passionate about her job. Her own experiences in life allow her to have this amazing compassion, support, and gentle guidance for her clients and their families. During her first year of work, she received a Rookie of the Year/Most Valuable New Employee award and was promoted to supervisor. She was offered a new job with higher pay and better benefits, but her current job is fighting to keep her. She plans to go on to get her PhD. She is supporting her four children and is now an amazing mother, able to help them deal with their father's death. She is beginning to let people in, to speak up about her illness, and to teach others what helps and what doesn't. What amazes us the most is Loni's desire to be an instrument of change for others with mental illness, others whose hearts grieve and ache for the loss of their loved ones and for loved ones who may not understand or know how to be supportive.

We have the responsibility to do this work and share it with you. Without fulfilling our mission, Loni might be dead and her children orphaned.

BRAIN WARRIOR MICHAEL PETERSON

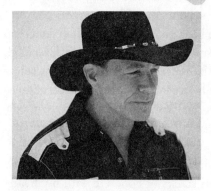

In 1997 country singer Michael Peterson was named *Billboard*'s Male Artist of the Year. He is known for such blockbuster songs as "From Here to Eternity," "Drink, Swear, Steal & Lie," and "Too Good to Be True." But after fifteen years on the road, his health was in noticeable decline: "Somehow over the course of my life, I had become numb to the messages that my body was sending me. . . . I didn't really notice until it got pretty severe." After late-night shows, changes in time and schedule, eating on the go, and regular encounters with unfamiliar beds, he knew that he didn't feel good. Life on the road had put him under an enormous amount of daily stress. He was 50 to 60 pounds overweight and had a difficult time staying alert in the afternoons on any given day. He found sleeping difficult and often woke feeling tired and unrested, plus he struggled with indigestion, plantar fasciitis, and a horrible backache.

By 2012 Michael decided it was time to get healthy. "The more in touch I got, the more I realized just how insane my old ways were." Michael and his wife found Daniel's book *Change Your Brain, Change Your Life* and decided to come to our clinic for evaluations that included SPECT scans. Michael explained how learning about his brain changed everything in his life:

"The simple awareness, that when you put garbage into your system, it affects your brain. It's not just that you are going to gain a few pounds. It's the whole idea of brain envy. For the first time in my life I became more passionate about brain health than being able to fit into a size of pants."

Michael's scan showed clear evidence of traumatic brain injury. When we asked him about it, he said he'd played football in high school as an offensive and defensive lineman and in college as an offensive lineman, and starting in his mid-twenties he got into breaking bricks with his head. In fact, he held the world record for it, once breaking thirty-four bricks at a time (see photo on page 248).

"Excuse me," Daniel said. "Can you say that again?"

Michael had joined a group of athletes who were involved with youth evangelism. The appeal of the group was based on athletes performing feats of strength to draw a crowd and share their testimonies of faith. They often performed four to five school assembly programs per day. One of Michael's stunts was to use his head to break through concrete bricks. The stacks were small at first, three to five bricks, which seemed easy enough at the time. Over time he started adding bricks to the stack and it became sort of a competition between Michael and the other guys on the team to see who could break the most. He said, "We were in our mid-twenties and still feeling 10-feet-tall and bulletproof." Eventually, he surpassed everyone else and at one point broke just short of 5 feet of concrete with one strike from his head. "I would bet in those twenty years I broke well over a thousand stacks of concrete with my head, maybe close to two thousand." One night in Tomball, Texas, the bricks did not break and he wound up with compression fractures in his neck and upper spine.

Michael wrote to us later, "Between high school and college football and twenty years of breaking concrete with my head there were many, many impacts to my skull. I suspect that some of the difficulties I have experienced in my life are easily traceable back to these chronic patterns of misuse of my skull. From where I sit now I would strongly urge any young person to avoid playing a sport where their head is going to be hit repeatedly, and I would never recommend anyone to break concrete with their head. It sounds silly even saying that. . . . But it didn't seem like a big deal at the time."

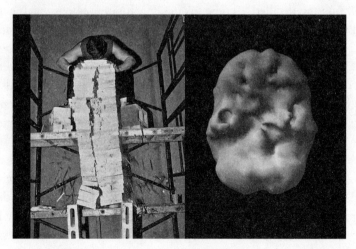

Seeing his scan caused Michael to become deeply committed to brain health. He became a Brain Warrior and completely changed his life. Michael is truly living a brain healthy lifestyle and has reached his goal of not having foggy-headed moments throughout the day. Not only has he transformed his own life but he also uses his public platform as a country music star to help others. Michael engages with adults and middle and high school students as an inspirational speaker promoting personal accountability, brain health, and the practice of gratitude as keys to overcoming adversity and achieving success in life. Michael feels a deep level of responsibility to teach others what he has learned.

He recently told us, "Having a Brain Warrior partner made a *huge* difference for me.

"My wife's commitment to my well-being was second only to her own. Watching her become a Brain Warrior continues to both challenge and inspire me. If you don't have a partner, consider becoming a partner for someone you love. It is amazing what determination arises in you when you are passionately attempting to help others.

"My last piece of counsel: We are all creatures of habit. There is a quote from Og Mandino I recite to myself every day, especially when I feel an old way of eating enticing me:

"'The only difference between those who have failed and those who have succeeded lies in the difference of their habits. Good habits are the key to all success. Bad habits are the unlocked door to failure.'

"I have followed the Amens' advice over and over these past few

MICHAEL'S BEFORE AND AFTER SCANS

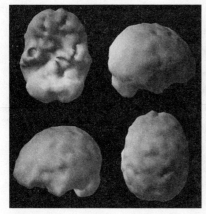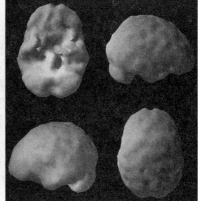

Before

After
Overall improved blood flow

years, and these choices have become my new habits. I intend to continue succeeding. Nothing is worth protecting more than my health. That's why I think the phrase 'Brain Warrior' is so appropriate. Tell me, what is more worth fighting for than your health? I have been transformed from a Brain 'Worry'er' to a 'Brain Warrior.'"

You can learn more about Michael's work at www.MichaelPeter sonOnline.com.

BRAIN WARRIOR DAVE ASPREY

After reading *Change Your Brain, Change Your Life*, Dave Asprey, CEO of Bulletproof, got a brain SPECT scan in 2003, and it changed everything in his life. In his words, "The SPECT scan rocked my world. I was a high-performing engineer, working full-time at a start-up that we sold for $600 million. At the same time I was getting an MBA from Wharton but was really struggling. I would sit down to do a test and I would get 100 percent on the first question, 50 percent on the next one, and I couldn't remember my name by the third question. I felt really guilty and knew something was wrong with me. I ended up being allowed to have extra time for tests, but still struggled. I barely graduated.

"After I read your book I decided to get a SPECT scan. The psychiatrist who evaluated it said, 'Dave, inside your brain there's total chaos—I don't know how you're standing here in front of me.' This led me to say, 'It's not me. It's my biology.' I had something that could be fixed or repaired and went from feeling that I was lazy, just wasn't trying hard enough, or was a bad person to being someone who had a medical issue that could and would be dealt with."

It turned out that Dave had been exposed to toxic mold in his home. After he underwent healing protocols, he became a warrior for his brain's health. When Dave saw his brain his relationship with it changed forever.

In his words, "My relationship with my brain changed a lot because I don't identify myself as being my brain. And, to this day, when something happens that I don't like or isn't like me, I think, 'What did my brain do?' not 'What did I do?' And there is a profound difference, because I can control what my brain does, but I am not my brain. For me it was a huge thing because it allowed me to be more forgiving of myself. And also, when I look at other people, I ask myself, is that person actually an evil person? Or is that a person who's profoundly toxic, or someone who has been abused or who whacked their head too many times, and they're acting that way without their own knowledge or consent, without their own permission? There's so much of that behavior in the world around me and around us, but people aren't aware of it; their medical professionals aren't aware of it—their psychologists, their spouses, their children—so there's a lot of people feeling terribly guilty about things they've done, who don't know there's a biological basis for their behavior. It's not a personality defect. I am living proof that the brain can be healed with the right strategies."

Dave took responsibility for his life and the lives of those he loves. He went on to produce *Moldy: The Toxic Mold Movie*, the first ever documentary about toxic mold, showing that hidden toxic mold in your home or work may be making you sick and impacting your performance every day, and what to do about it.

BRAIN WARRIOR SHERYL

Common to many girls with attention deficit disorder, no one noticed that Sheryl struggled in school with focus, organization, and impulse control. Due to her struggles, as a teenager she began to feel anxious and started having migraine headaches, for which she was prescribed anti-anxiety medication as well as medications for her headaches varying from antidepressants to pain relievers. In high school, as a way to fit in and medicate her own pain she started drinking and doing drugs on weekends to excess, not realizing she was teaching her brain how to "deal" with uncomfortable feelings. This started a long downward spiral that included multiple suicide attempts, hospitalizations, counseling, medications, and a variety of attempts to figure out exactly how to deal with life. She felt as though she could not function in this world . . . She must have "broken her brain." The more she tried to fix it, the worse her life became. In her mind, the drugs and alcohol were the solution, not the problem. That was the only time there was a sense of reprieve and the ability to take a deep breath. At one point she was taking 220 milligrams of OxyContin and 6 milligrams of Klonopin prescribed for the anxiety and headaches. Yet when you add a few terrible marriages, divorces, twenty to thirty moves, a job change, and a custody battle, she had more problems than she could handle. Even if she stopped digging at this point, the hole was too deep.

After a suicide attempt by drug overdose she was taken to an emergency room, where Sheryl's father looked at her and said, "Your eyes are dead." When he said those words she could see how devastated he was, and it crushed her. Her solution to her problems was causing more pain to those she loved. Because she couldn't figure out how to stop hurting the people she loved, she still wanted to die. Her life was such a mess and if she could not handle it with "drugs as the solution," how was she ever going to handle it without them?

After a few days in the hospital with the drugs cleared out of her system, she looked in the mirror and saw what her father was talking about. "I looked like I had the life choked out of me. I was 95 pounds at five foot seven and forty-five years old. I literally said to myself (and God), 'Well, this is quite a conundrum! I can't die (I'm on suicide watch) and I don't know how to live! Now what?!'"

She immediately felt her answer. For the first time in a long time—maybe ever—she felt as though things were going to be okay. "It felt like I received a hug from God," she said. "Through a series of thoughts and prayers, and reading Proverbs, I realized God works through people, and I started to ask people for help, and taking suggestions. I was taught how to eat an elephant: One bite at a time. So, I started chewing."

She also started looking for answers as to how and why she ended up where she was. Sheryl describes herself as an intelligent, kind, and caring individual, so she was baffled. "How could I get here?"

After inpatient treatment, she was concerned about the ten medications she had been put on to stabilize her brain and decided to stop them to gain a sense of her baseline functioning. During this time, she saw Daniel's PBS program *Change Your Brain, Change Your Life* and bought his books, including *Healing ADD*, and was "totally over the moon" with the research, discoveries, and explanations. It literally was a life changer.

Armed with new information, Sheryl's life began changing in many, many ways. In her own words, Sheryl told us, "I went from being homeless, hopeless, and helpless; on disability; unemployable; divorced three times, without custody of my three children; and did not have one person I felt I could call to save my life. Today, I am fifty-one years old, employed as an RN, BSN on a busy cardio-surgical-trauma unit at a hospital, and I also teach classes on substance-abuse-treatment-related issues at an institute for addiction counseling. I am in a stable relationship, and most important, I am able to be a good mother, daughter, friend, employee, and sponsor. My parents are proud of me, and what a gift it is to be able to bring them joy instead of pain and fear. . . . Knowledge is power. This new knowledge gave me the 'why' and 'how' I broke my brain, which meant I could also fix it. That knowledge is a gift that saved my life."

Sheryl told us, "Your revelations have not only changed my brain and my life but also had a ripple effect. I am able to share what I have learned with clients, patients, students, friends, family, and my children. I am a Brain Warrior for life."

Six plus years after Sheryl became sober she came to Amen Clinics for a SPECT scan. It looked so much better than she thought it would. She was told, "You have a *beautiful* cerebellum!" Her brain was no longer broken. Her new behavior caused her brain to heal.

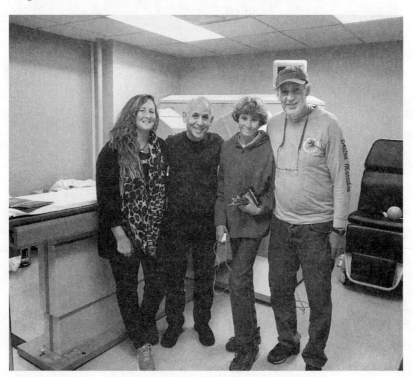

Sheryl, Daniel and Her Family at Amen Clinics, New York City

Brain Warrior Responsibilities Takeaways

Brain Warriors are serious, relentless, and responsible.

Your life is not just about you; it is about generations of you, literally.

Leave epigenetic marks that are healthy for your children and grandchildren.

Once you know this information, you are responsible to plant it in your life, so it can grow in the lives of those you influence.

Change in others may not happen right away. Sometimes it might even take decades.

You speak your love to your children and grandchildren by your actions today.

You are contagious to others.

Others are contagious to you.

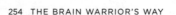

PART 7

Yearlong Brain Warrior Basic Training

Starts with the 14-Day Brain Boost

This moment contains all moments.

—C. S. LEWIS, *THE GREAT DIVORCE*

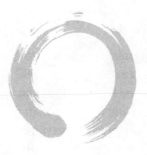

NOW IS THE TIME

C. S. Lewis's powerful allegory *The Great Divorce* describes a bus ride from hell toward heaven and highlights that hell is in the minds of people who keep themselves trapped in short-term thinking, excuses, and blaming others for their circumstances as a way of living.

In one of the book's most powerful scenes, an unsubstantial, ghostlike figure at a bus stop had a red lizard on his shoulder who was whispering things in his ear that alternately made him angry, then amused him. The lizard represents the voices in our heads that diminish us, then give us permission to do the wrong things that damage our health and lives. The ghost decided that the lizard's nonsense was inappropriate for the journey and was on his way back to the bus to go back home, when he was approached by a large, bright humanlike figure—an angel—who said, "Off so soon?"

After a brief discussion, the angel asked the ghost if he would like him to quiet the lizard and the ghost said yes. The ghost made a tentative decision to change, to move his life forward without the negative chatter in his head that was holding him back. But when the angel's hands got close to kill the lizard, the ghost quickly backtracked, making excuse after excuse: "You're burning me. . . . Keep away. . . . There's time to discuss it later. . . . You don't have to kill the lizard. . . . He's quiet now. . . . I'll run back by tonight's bus and get an opinion from my own doctor."

The angel replied to each of the excuses, "I never said it wouldn't hurt you. I said it wouldn't kill you. . . . There is no time. . . . The gradual process is of no use at all. . . . This moment contains all moments. I cannot kill it against your will. May I have your permission?"

When the ghost finally made the decision to change, despite the potential pain, he transformed quickly into a strong, newly made man; the lizard, once dead, also transformed into a powerful stallion that took his owner toward heaven.

Breaking free of the chains of the past requires
a clear decision that now *is the time to get*
healthy.
Not tomorrow.
Not Monday.
Not next week.
Not January 2.
Not when you are finally sick of feeling sick.
But right now, *this very minute.*

In our experience, when you commit to now, *you stop looking for short-cuts and excuses and you change your life in a powerful way.* Making the decision to change at a deep emotional level and getting rid of the excuses that keep illness in your life—such as "I'll start after the holidays"—is the first step in becoming a lasting Brain Warrior. Then it is boldly planting the program into your life, step by step, over an extended period of time—for at least a year. The allure of ten-day, two-week, thirty-day programs is powerful, but they rarely change anyone for the long term, because they have a short-term mind-set. Here's one of the best examples of the negative consequences of short-term thinking.

During one of our appearances on public television we worked with a local host who looked amazing compared to the last time we had seen him. We asked what he was doing to lose weight. He told us he was on the human chorionic gonadotropin (hCG) diet, which consisted of being injected regularly with the pregnancy hormone hCG, combined with eating 500 calories per day in twenty-six-day cycles. He had lost 30 pounds, and it showed. But as he was telling us about his diet, he said he was just finishing the last cycle and had ordered two deep-dish pizzas from his favorite Italian restaurant in Chicago as a way to celebrate. As he said the last sentence we must have had horrified looks on our faces.

"What?" he asked.

Daniel said, "It is like you just got out of an alcohol rehab center and as a way to celebrate you are going to get drunk!"

The next time we saw him he had put back on all of the weight. Then several years later, he decided to make a lifetime decision to focus on his health and has kept the weight off and now looks amazing.

The Brain Warrior's Way is a program to get control of your brain and your body for the rest of your life and help you revitalize your health now and for generations to come. As such, it *requires continual engagement for at least a year so it becomes part of the fabric of your mind, habits, and everyday life.* Old bad habits are not going to be broken in a few weeks, as many books would have you believe, and new habits are not sustained for the long term until you create and strengthen the underlying neural networks that help you make good decisions. Just like mastering the piano, elevating your golf game, or becoming a wise investor require training over time, you too need consistent effort over time to become a Brain Warrior for life. An added benefit of being focused on this program for a full year is that you'll actually be able to keep the lost weight off. Yearlong healthy habits help reset and normalize one of the main hormones involved with appetite.[154]

GET STARTED NOW: THE 14-DAY BRAIN BOOST

To begin, we have developed a plan to get you started with a big win. We call it the 14-Day Brain Boost. We realize in order for you to stay motivated to live the Brain Warrior's Way you must start to feel better quickly.

If you do the program as we outline in this section—without cheating—you can look forward to the following benefits in just two weeks:

- Disappearance of carbohydrate and sugar cravings within three to seven days
- Reduction of joint pain or swelling in your body as a result of decreased inflammation
- Dramatic improvement in digestion and any digestion-related problems you may have
- Skin that is clearer and noticeably more vibrant
- Improved ability to focus
- Improved mood and sense of inner peace
- Increased energy
- Losing 5, to as much as 15, pounds, if needed

You can feel better in a very short period of time if you just do what we ask. Do it all to get the best results. We challenge you to fourteen days. You can do anything for fourteen days and in that time you can start to build new habits and remodel your taste buds to enjoy wholesome, life-affirming foods, rather than craving the artificially flavored, addictive ones. And in fourteen days you can dramatically improve your energy, focus, and mental clarity, and begin to heal your gut, rosacea, and chronic pain. Feeling better quickly will boost your confidence and motivation.

GET PREPARED

1. Make a decision now to commit to the plan for fourteen days.
2. Get your mind right. There is no suffering required or recommended. This program is about abundance and not deprivation; that's why it's critical to have the right mind-set.
3. Make an appointment with your health-care provider to get your important numbers checked right away. If you do not have a health-care provider or he or she will not order the tests, you can go to websites like SaveOnLabs (saveonlabs.com) and order them for yourself. Your doctor is not your mother, father, or boss. He or she should be your partner in healthcare.
4. If you snore, stop breathing at night, or are chronically tired during the day, get assessed for sleep apnea immediately.
5. Every day take a multiple vitamin and omega-3 fatty acid supplement. Make sure you know and optimize your vitamin D level and take supplements geared toward your brain type (see Part 2). You can discover your brain type by taking our free Brain Health Assessment at amenclinics. com.
6. Every day complete the 14-Day Brain Warrior's Way Journal, found in this chapter and online at mybrainfitlife. com. This is a critical step to accelerated mindfulness and being successful. If you continue this after fourteen days it will continue to boost your success.

7. Clean out your pantry and all the devious places you hide low-quality food: elsewhere in your home, at work, or in your car. Remove all the foods that hurt you and keep the ones that help you. (More detailed instructions can be found in *The Brain Warrior's Way Cookbook*.)

8. Routines will help you succeed. The more you can get into a groove, the easier the program becomes. Find five breakfasts, lunches, dinners, snacks, and desserts you like. Find the same time each day to work out.

9. Pick a buddy with whom to do the program. Our research suggests people double the program's effectiveness if they do it with at least one other person.

10. Make sleep a priority!

CLEAN YOUR PANTRY: DITCH THESE FOODS

- Bread, pasta, tortillas, and other foods containing gluten
- Sugary breakfast cereals
- Condiments—such as ketchup, soy sauce, and barbecue sauce—that contain sugar, artificial ingredients, or gluten
- Products containing corn, including popcorn, cornbread, and popped corn chips
- Processed dairy foods, such as cow's milk, cheese, cream, yogurt, and ice cream
- Foods that contain high-fructose corn syrup or trans (hydrogenated) fats
- Foods that contain sugar, artificial sweeteners, or soy
- Fruit juice (even 100 percent fresh!)
- Grain-based foods, such as rice, instant oatmeal, wheat, barley, and rye
- Jams, jellies, and pancake syrup
- Cooking oils that contain corn, safflower, canola, soy, and vegetable oils
- Processed frozen dinners
- Processed meats, such as hot dogs

(CONTINUED)

- Processed snacks, including potato chips, popcorn, pretzels, tortilla chips, and crackers
- Soy-based foods, such as protein bars, powders, and snack foods
- Sugary processed snacks, such as cake, cookies, cupcakes, and candy
- Sweetened drinks, such as fruit punch, lemonade, and soda
- White potatoes

YOUR 14-DAY MEAL PLAN

Enjoy the following meals for fourteen days and forever after. (We eat this way 95 percent of the time.) Start each day with 16 to 20 ounces of water and drink water throughout the day. Enjoy any of the foods designated as the Best 100 Brain Foods listed in Part 3. Here are some great examples of meals you can have from *The Brain Warrior's Way Cookbook*. You can also find these recipes and many more online at mybrainfitlife.com.

BREAKFAST

Super-Focus Smoothie
Cherry Mint Blast
Coconut Berry Cooler
Muffin Tin Egg Frittatas
Omega Egg Burrito to Go
Spanish Scramble

LUNCH OR DINNER

SALADS

Savory Grapefruit Avocado Salad
Orange, Fennel, and Blueberry Salad
Kale and Quinoa Tabbouleh
Wilted Kale and Strawberry Salad
Cashew Kale Salad with Chicken

Creamy Coconut Curry Soup
Cream of Asparagus Soup
Healing Chicken Herb Soup
Lentil Vegetable Soup

PROTEIN

Creamy Pesto Halibut
Fresh and Tangy Trout
Rosemary Thyme Chicken
Chicken Asada
Herb Roasted Rack of Lamb (Daniel's all-time favorite)

VEGGIES

Cruciferous Cold Slaw
Peppery Bok Choy
Grilled asparagus
Steamed broccoli
Roasted mixed vegetables

SNACKS

One-Minute Avocado Egg Basket
Quick Egg Salad Wrap
Snappy Chicken Salad Snacks
Coconut Avocado Protein Pudding
Chopped veggies with guacamole or hummus

DESSERT

Go light with dessert. Choose from this list for the first two weeks and consume only small portions.

Fresh Berries with Macadamia Cream Sauce
Chocolate Protein Sorbet
Sweet Potato Coconut Flan

Choose one of these per day:
    Brain in Love Bars
    Brain on Joy Bars
    Two-Ingredient Nutty Butter Cups

FOR FOURTEEN DAYS, AND FOREVER AFTER IF YOU ARE REALLY SERIOUS ABOUT BRAIN HEALTH

Eliminate These Foods

Sugar, in all forms
High-glycemic, low-fiber foods (bread, white potatoes, rice, pasta)
All fruit juices
Grains (may be reintroduced after two weeks, but only in small amounts as a condiment)
Processed foods
Artificial colors and sweeteners
Food additives
Agave
Gluten (wheat, barley, rye, spelt, faro)
Soy
Corn
Creamed veggies
Dairy products
Peanuts
Certain oils, such as canola, peanut, vegetable, corn, safflower, and sunflower oils

Limit These Foods

Alcohol: no more than 4 normal-size glasses per week (a normal-size glass of alcohol is considered 1 ounce of hard liquor, 6 ounces of wine, or 8 ounces of beer)
Caffeine: no more than 150 milligrams a day, which is one 12-ounce cup of coffee or three 12-ounce cups of green tea

The 14-Day Brain Warrior's Way Journal

DAY 1: DEVELOP LASTING HABITS

Motivation Blast: The war for your health is won between your ears.

What is my goal today?

_____

_____

_____

_____

Three things I am grateful for today

1. _____

2. _____

3. _____

Whom shall I appreciate today?

_____

_____

Today's Weight _____ Hours Slept _____

On a scale of 1 to 10 rate the following (1 = poor, 10 = great)

Mood ____ Energy ____ Focus ____
Memory ____ Inner peace ____ Decision making ____

Choose five brain healthy habits from the following list to do today

❏ Read my One Page Miracle

❏ Start the day with 16 to 20 ounces of water (8 to 10 ounces for kids)

- ❏ Focus on eating healthy without cheating
- ❏ Eat brain healthy snacks, maintain stable blood sugar
- ❏ Engage in smart exercise (bursting, weight training, coordination exercises)
- ❏ Learn something new
- ❏ Combat stress (hypnosis, meditation, brain-enhancing music)
- ❏ Learn from at least one mistake
- ❏ Get 7 to 8 hours of sleep
- ❏ Practice good decision making
- ❏ Take my supplements
- ❏ Connect with a Brain Warrior buddy
- ❏ Kill the ANTs

The Brain Warrior's Way Journal

DAY 1: BRAIN-ENHANCING FOOD

TIME	FOOD AND BEVERAGE	HEALTHY (YES OR NO)
	Breakfast	
	Snack	
	Lunch	
	Snack	
	Dinner	
	Other	

The Brain Warrior's Way Journal

DAY 2: DEVELOP LASTING HABITS

Motivation Blast: The greatest wealth is health.—Virgil

What is my goal today?

_____

_____

_____

_____

Three things I am grateful for today

1. _____

2. _____

3. _____

Whom shall I appreciate today?

_____

_____

Today's Weight _____ Hours Slept _____

On a scale of 1 to 10 rate the following (1 = poor, 10 = great)

Mood ____ Energy ____ Focus ____
Memory ____ Inner peace ____ Decision making ____

Choose five brain healthy habits from the following list to do today

❑ Read my One Page Miracle

❑ Start the day with 16 to 20 ounces of water (8 to 10 ounces for kids)

- ❏ Focus on eating healthy without cheating
- ❏ Eat brain healthy snacks, maintain stable blood sugar
- ❏ Engage in smart exercise (bursting, weight training, coordination exercises)
- ❏ Learn something new
- ❏ Combat stress (hypnosis, meditation, brain-enhancing music)
- ❏ Learn from at least one mistake
- ❏ Get 7 to 8 hours of sleep
- ❏ Practice good decision making
- ❏ Take my supplements
- ❏ Connect with a Brain Warrior buddy
- ❏ Kill the ANTs

The Brain Warrior's Way Journal

DAY 2: BRAIN-ENHANCING FOOD

TIME	FOOD AND BEVERAGE	HEALTHY (YES OR NO)
	Breakfast	
	Snack	
	Lunch	
	Snack	
	Dinner	
	Other	

DANIEL'S BRAIN WARRIOR ROUTINE:
PURPOSE, SLEEP, EXERCISE, AND FOOD

Sleep

Start with 7 to 8 hours of sleep, even when I travel. I try never to take flights before 10:00 A.M. to make sure I get enough sleep.

Exercise

Wear a Fitbit to keep me on track, aiming for 10,000 steps a day.

Work out with a trainer twice a week, lifting weights and stretching.

Work out with my father once or twice a week to keep him strong, but I benefit too—socially, emotionally, and physically.

Walk as if I were late, with bursts, three to four times a week.

Food (Try to Never Let Myself Get Hungry)

Start the day with water and Tana's Pumpkin Spice Cappuccino (Amazing! See recipe in *The Brain Warrior's Way Cookbook*)

Breakfast

One of Tana's Breakfast Shakes *or* stir-fried eggs with veggies

Snack

Chopped veggies with hummus or mashed avocados

Lunch

Salad with protein and veggies, vinegar and olive oil dressing on the side (put vinegar on the salad first to not overdo the oil) or a stir-fry with protein and lots of veggies, without rice or bread (this allows my energy to stay high all afternoon)

Brain on Joy Bar for a treat (this is a chocolate-coconut bar we make that is 160 calories and has no sugar or dairy)

Late-Afternoon Snack

100-calorie pack of nuts

(CONTINUED)

Dinner

Salad

Protein: fish, chicken, lamb, pork, or steak

Veggies: braised cauliflower, Brussels sprouts, or broccoli

Occasional sweet potato or quinoa

Dessert: one of Tana's dessert creations on occasion

Fast for 12 hours from dinner to breakfast.

I eat this way 95 percent of the time. I also do not drink alcohol, because I don't really enjoy the taste and don't see the benefit. I like having my wits about me all the time.

My relaxation is spending time with my children, grandchildren, parents, or friends; exercising; watching movies; or writing.

The Brain Warrior's Way Journal

Motivation Blast: Who has more fun? The person with the good brain or the one with the bad brain?

What is my goal today?

_____

_____

_____

_____

Three things I am grateful for today

1. _____

2. _____

3. _____

Whom shall I appreciate today?

_____

_____

Today's Weight _____ Hours Slept _____

On a scale of 1 to 10 rate the following (1 = poor, 10 = great)

Mood ____ Energy ____ Focus ____
Memory ____ Inner peace ____ Decision making ____

Choose five brain healthy habits from the following list to do today

❏ Read my One Page Miracle

❏ Start the day with 16 to 20 ounces of water (8 to 10 ounces for kids)

- ❏ Focus on eating healthy without cheating
- ❏ Eat brain healthy snacks, maintain stable blood sugar
- ❏ Engage in smart exercise (bursting, weight training, coordination exercises)
- ❏ Learn something new
- ❏ Combat stress (hypnosis, meditation, brain-enhancing music)
- ❏ Learn from at least one mistake
- ❏ Get 7 to 8 hours of sleep
- ❏ Practice good decision making
- ❏ Take my supplements
- ❏ Connect with a Brain Warrior buddy
- ❏ Kill the ANTs

The Brain Warrior's Way Journal

DAY 3: BRAIN-ENHANCING FOOD

TIME	FOOD AND BEVERAGE	HEALTHY (YES OR NO)
Breakfast		
Snack		
Lunch		
Snack		
Dinner		
Other		

SIMPLE TIPS TO GET STARTED

Keep these strategies in mind as you plan your meals each day:

- Eat breakfast within 1 hour of waking up and eat every 3 to 4 hours by having either a meal or snack, so you are eating five or six times a day.
- Limit foods that are overprocessed and overcooked. Instead, opt for as many raw and lightly cooked choices as possible.
- Shake hands with protein. When measuring aids are unavailable, use the palm of your hand to determine a good portion size for protein foods. A 20- to 40-gram serving of meat or fish is about the size and width of the palm of your hand.
- If you are going to cheat, do it with protein and healthy fat, *not carbohydrates!* This will send satisfying signals to your brain, unlike simple carbs, which make you hungrier.
- Instead of bread, use lettuce wraps for sandwiches and burgers.
- Never allow yourself to become too hungry. This is the key to avoiding self-sabotage and cheating. That's why we want you to eat something every 3 to 4 hours initially.
- If you continue to feel hungry between meals, increase your intake of raw or lightly cooked (nonstarchy) vegetables— they're "free" foods, and you can have as much as you want. Keep in mind, though, that fruit, with its high concentration of fructose (fruit sugar), raises blood sugar and insulin levels and should be limited to one or two servings a day.
- Stay hydrated. This will help curb hunger and improve the quality of your decisions.
- Plan ahead. Do your menu planning, shopping, and food preparation in advance. We use one day each week to prepare for the following days. Pack your lunch and have plenty of nutritious snacks on hand, along with an ice chest that's ready to go whenever you leave the house. The better prepared you can be, the more successful you will be. As the saying goes, if you fail to plan, you plan to fail.
- Always prepare extra food when cooking and pack leftovers for the next day's lunch.

- Always have hummus and fresh avocados handy for guacamole.
- Never let a waiter leave bread on the table when dining out.
- Have a list of delicious alternatives handy for the foods you will be eliminating.

The Brain Warrior's Way Journal

DAY 4: DEVELOP LASTING HABITS

Motivation Blast: This moment contains all moments. Now is the time to get healthy.

What is my goal today?

_____

_____

_____

_____

Three things I am grateful for today

1. _____

2. _____

3. _____

Whom shall I appreciate today?

_____

_____

Today's Weight _____ Hours Slept _____

On a scale of 1 to 10 rate the following (1 = poor, 10 = great)

Mood _____ Energy _____ Focus _____
Memory _____ Inner peace _____ Decision making _____

Choose five brain healthy habits from the following list to do today

❑ Read my One Page Miracle

❑ Start the day with 16 to 20 ounces of water (8 to 10 ounces for kids)

- ❏ Focus on eating healthy without cheating
- ❏ Eat brain healthy snacks, maintain stable blood sugar
- ❏ Engage in smart exercise (bursting, weight training, coordination exercises)
- ❏ Learn something new
- ❏ Combat stress (hypnosis, meditation, brain-enhancing music)
- ❏ Learn from at least one mistake
- ❏ Get 7 to 8 hours of sleep
- ❏ Practice good decision making
- ❏ Take my supplements
- ❏ Connect with a Brain Warrior buddy
- ❏ Kill the ANTs

The Brain Warrior's Way Journal

DAY 4: BRAIN-ENHANCING FOOD

TIME	FOOD AND BEVERAGE	HEALTHY (YES OR NO)
	Breakfast	
	Snack	
	Lunch	
	Snack	
	Dinner	
	Other	

CREATE A PATTERN INTERRUPT

Cravings are likely to become less frequent and less intense as you gain skill as a Brain Warrior. However, they may still occur on occasion, usually when you least expect them. We always want you armed with a plan! A "pattern interrupt" is a strategy that disrupts your focus from whatever triggered your craving. Make a list of simple things that can be quickly executed when a yearning for junk strikes. Some of our favorite options include these:

Going for a walk

Drinking a tall glass of water or a cup of green tea

Eating a plate of veggies

Calling a friend

Taking a shower

Listening to brain healthy music

Going for a drive

If you're home, simply getting out of the house (and away from your temptation) usually does the trick.

If you find yourself giving in occasionally, you need a second strategy to get back on track quickly. Remember, there is no failing, only quitting. Our backup strategy is to be conscious as we engage in making a choice that is less than optimal. Don't be a zombie and mechanically polish off a quart of ice cream. Own your actions. Also, follow the three-bite rule and enjoy those first three bites. It's the first three bites that give you the pleasure hit. If you stop at three bites you're less likely to trigger the inflammation and hormones that in turn trigger addiction. Then get rid of whatever's left (get it out of the house) and move forward. Taking three mindful bites is better than going on a mindless zombie binge.

The Brain Warrior's Way Journal

DAY 5: DEVELOPING LASTING HABITS

Motivation Blast: Don't believe every stupid thought you have.

What is my goal today?

_____

_____

_____

_____

Three things I am grateful for today

1. _____

2. _____

3. _____

Whom shall I appreciate today?

_____

_____

Today's Weight _____ Hours Slept _____

On a scale of 1 to 10 rate the following (1 = poor, 10 = great)

Mood ____ Energy ____ Focus ____
Memory ____ Inner peace ____ Decision making ____

Choose five brain healthy habits from the following list to do today

❏ Read my One Page Miracle

❏ Start the day with 16 to 20 ounces of water (8 to 10 ounces for kids)

- ❏ Focus on eating healthy without cheating
- ❏ Eat brain healthy snacks, maintain stable blood sugar
- ❏ Engage in smart exercise (bursting, weight training, coordination exercises)
- ❏ Learn something new
- ❏ Combat stress (hypnosis, meditation, brain-enhancing music)
- ❏ Learn from at least one mistake
- ❏ Get 7 to 8 hours of sleep
- ❏ Practice good decision making
- ❏ Take my supplements
- ❏ Connect with a Brain Warrior buddy
- ❏ Kill the ANTs

The Brain Warrior's Way Journal

DAY 5: BRAIN-ENHANCING FOOD

TIME	FOOD AND BEVERAGE	HEALTHY (YES OR NO)
	Breakfast	
	Snack	
	Lunch	
	Snack	
	Dinner	
	Other	

SIMPLE SWAPS FOR SUCCESS

As you wean yourself off unhealthful foods, use these super swap strategies:

- Drink green tea or herbal tea with a few drops of stevia instead of coffee. Our favorite "comfort drink" is sugar-free, steamed almond milk with a bag of green chai tea and a few drops of cinnamon-flavored stevia. This is a guilt-free tea latte.
- Use a little light coconut milk in your tea or coffee instead of half-and-half or soy creamer.
- Drink sparkling water sweetened with root beer–flavored stevia instead of diet soda.
- Squeeze lemon or lime juice or a few drops of lemon-flavored stevia into seltzer, and drink it instead of wine. This is a great drink for parties when you want a drink to be social but don't want to consume alcohol.
- Enjoy sugar-free almond milk instead of dairy milk or soy milk.
- Replace candy with our Brain on Joy bars. They taste exactly like chocolate-coconut candy, but they are sweetened with stevia and erythritol. This is a great alternative when you are craving chocolate, but they should still be eaten only as a treat. The recipe can be found at brainmdhealth.com.
- Replace ice cream with Chocolate Protein Sorbet (see the *Brain Warrior's Way Cookbook*).
- Eat half an apple with almond butter instead of cookies and candy.
- Eat a quarter cup of raw unsalted nuts and one piece of 70 percent cocoa dark chocolate instead of muffins, candies, and cookies.

The Brain Warrior's Way Journal

DAY 6: DEVELOPING LASTING HABITS

Motivation Blast: Getting truly well is about abundance, never deprivation.

What is my goal today?

_____

_____

_____

_____

Three things I am grateful for today

1. _____

2. _____

3. _____

Whom shall I appreciate today?

_____

_____

Today's Weight _____ Hours Slept _____

On a scale of 1 to 10 rate the following (1 = poor, 10 = great)

Mood ___ Energy ___ Focus ___
Memory ___ Inner peace ___ Decision making ___

Choose five brain healthy habits from the following list to do today

❏ Read my One Page Miracle

❏ Start the day with 16 to 20 ounces of water (8 to 10 ounces for kids)

- ❑ Focus on eating healthy without cheating
- ❑ Eat brain healthy snacks, maintain stable blood sugar
- ❑ Engage in smart exercise (bursting, weight training, coordination exercises)
- ❑ Learn something new
- ❑ Combat stress (hypnosis, meditation, brain-enhancing music)
- ❑ Learn from at least one mistake
- ❑ Get 7 to 8 hours of sleep
- ❑ Practice good decision making
- ❑ Take my supplements
- ❑ Connect with a Brain Warrior buddy
- ❑ Kill the ANTs

The Brain Warrior's Way Journal

DAY 6: BRAIN-ENHANCING FOOD

TIME	FOOD AND BEVERAGE	HEALTHY (YES OR NO)
Breakfast		
Snack		
Lunch		
Snack		
Dinner		
Other		

BRAIN WARRIOR FAST FOOD—
SMOOTHIES

Smoothies are our favorite example of a perfectly balanced meal! They're convenient, delicious, and hydrating and a perfect way to optimize nutrition with a meal of protein, healthy fat, phytonutrients, vitamins, minerals, fiber, and other fabulous nutrients. And they're great for Brain Warriors on the run! Once you start making them, you'll wonder how you managed your busy life without them. Here are some simple tips for making sensational, power-packed smoothies.

- Use a high-powered blender. It doesn't have to be expensive, but it's best if it's high powered.
- Play with ingredients and be creative, but pay attention to sugar and calorie content. Make sure to include at least 1 tablespoon of healthy fat and 20 to 30 grams of protein.
- Athletes can use pure coconut water, which is God's natural electrolyte-rich sports drink, as a smoothie base. If you like to add ice to your smoothies, try freezing coconut water in an ice cube tray and toss coconut cubes into the blender instead of ice.
- Add soluble fiber, such as inulin (you can buy it in a powder form).
- Consider adding superfoods such as bee pollen, maca root powder, acai, pomegranate, and goji powder. Many are believed to have antioxidants or anti-inflammatory properties.
- Add freeze-dried greens, which contain lots of fruit and vegetable extracts. Be sure to check for the presence of gluten.
- Keep an eye on calories and nutritional content, especially sugar. The recipes in *The Brain Warrior's Way Cookbook* are a balance of protein, healthy fat, and an abundance of micronutrients and phytonutrients. Many smoothies, especially commercially made ones, are sugar bombs made with several pieces of fruit. That is a huge burst of sugar you don't need.

(CONTINUED)

- Raw greens contribute lots of fabulous nutrients to smoothies, but they have a bitter taste that can take some getting used to. If you are sensitive to the taste of raw greens, start with a small amount and gradually add more as you acquire a taste for them. Your goal should be three or four parts greens to one part fruit. You can also add 1 teaspoon of raw honey (if you are not insulin resistant) to soften the bitterness of the greens, but once you get used to the flavor of the greens, cut back the honey and eventually eliminate your use of sweeteners other than stevia.
- Raw cocoa is one of our favorite smoothie ingredients—it is the pure form of cocoa before it has been processed. It is loaded with antioxidants and phytonutrients and adds fun flavor. You can find it in most health food stores.
- Add 1 or 2 teaspoons of coconut butter or almond butter to add the appropriate amount of healthy fat, soften the taste of the greens, and add a creamy texture to your smoothie.
- Add 1 tablespoon of flaxseed, hemp seed, or chia seeds for fiber and plant-based proteins. They are high in omega-3 fatty acids and contain potent cancer-fighting properties. Do not use flax oil because it contains inflammatory omega-6 fatty acids and loses most of its anticancer benefits during processing.

The Brain Warrior's Way Journal

DAY 7: DEVELOPING LASTING HABITS

Motivation Blast: You are not stuck with the brain you have; you can make it better.

What is my goal today?

_____

_____

_____

_____

Three things I am grateful for today

1. _____

2. _____

3. _____

Whom shall I appreciate today?

_____

_____

Today's Weight _____ Hours Slept _____

On a scale of 1 to 10 rate the following (1 = poor, 10 = great)

Mood ____ Energy ____ Focus ____
Memory ____ Inner peace ____ Decision making ____

Choose five brain healthy habits from the following list to do today

❏ Read my One Page Miracle

❏ Start the day with 16 to 20 ounces of water (8 to 10 ounces for kids)

- ❏ Focus on eating healthy without cheating
- ❏ Eat brain healthy snacks, maintain stable blood sugar
- ❏ Engage in smart exercise (bursting, weight training, coordination exercises)
- ❏ Learn something new
- ❏ Combat stress (hypnosis, meditation, brain-enhancing music)
- ❏ Learn from at least one mistake
- ❏ Get 7 to 8 hours of sleep
- ❏ Practice good decision making
- ❏ Take my supplements
- ❏ Connect with a Brain Warrior buddy
- ❏ Kill the ANTs

The Brain Warrior's Way Journal

DAY 7: BRAIN-ENHANCING FOOD

TIME	FOOD AND BEVERAGE	HEALTHY (YES OR NO)
	Breakfast	
	Snack	
	Lunch	
	Snack	
	Dinner	
	Other	

NO LONGER CAPTIVE TO CARB CRAVINGS

There's a simple formula for breaking the addiction to sugar and simple carbs. It works like magic for most of our patients, but it's really chemistry and brain science. If you've been captive to carbs, follow these steps:

1. Eating small amounts of protein and healthful fats with each meal will begin to reset the hormones of metabolism. Protein is key, so don't go more than a few hours without eating a small amount of it. In fact, increasing your protein intake throughout the day will rev your metabolism and enhance weight loss—and tell your brain you're full.

2. Increase the volume of your meals and snacks by adding *lots* of vegetables (and a little fruit). This will increase fiber as well as hydration and will keep you full longer, satisfy your need to munch, and provide your body with super nutrition.

3. For the first two weeks, avoid grains completely. As you gain control over your dependence on sugar and simple carbs you'll be able to add certain grains back into your diet in small amounts—like a condiment. They should never be a staple. Eat no more than a half a cup at a time and not every day. Even though whole grains contain complex carbohydrates, they still eventually break down into sugar in your body. If you do choose to eat them, you can lessen their impact on your blood sugar by eating them with lean protein and healthy fats.

4. Remember, this is *not* deprivation. You are simply replacing, not erasing. Although you're eliminating bread, pasta, and other starchy foods that don't serve your health, you'll be eating other foods that do. Lean protein, vegetables, a bit of fruit, and healthy fats will do far more to nourish you and increase your feelings of satisfaction than sugar and simple carbs, once the addiction is under control.

5. Remember, animal foods are not the only source of protein. Nuts, seeds, vegetarian protein powders (be sure they're gluten free), and greens also add a significant amount of protein to your diet.

The Brain Warrior's Way Journal

DAY 8: DEVELOPING LASTING HABITS

Motivation Blast: Sheepdogs are serious, highly trained, and purpose-driven and love their sheep, even when the love is not returned.

What is my goal today?

_____

_____

_____

_____

Three things I am grateful for today

1. _____

2. _____

3. _____

Whom shall I appreciate today?

_____

_____

Today's Weight _____ Hours Slept _____

On a scale of 1 to 10 rate the following (1 = poor, 10 = great)

Mood ____ Energy ____ Focus ____
Memory ____ Inner peace ____ Decision making ____

Choose five brain healthy habits from the following list to do today

❑ Read my One Page Miracle

❑ Start the day with 16 to 20 ounces of water (8 to 10 ounces for kids)

- ❑ Focus on eating healthy without cheating
- ❑ Eat brain healthy snacks, maintain stable blood sugar
- ❑ Engage in smart exercise (bursting, weight training, coordination exercises)
- ❑ Learn something new
- ❑ Combat stress (hypnosis, meditation, brain-enhancing music)
- ❑ Learn from at least one mistake
- ❑ Get 7 to 8 hours of sleep
- ❑ Practice good decision making
- ❑ Take my supplements
- ❑ Connect with a Brain Warrior buddy
- ❑ Kill the ANTs

The Brain Warrior's Way Journal

DAY 8: BRAIN-ENHANCING FOOD

TIME	FOOD AND BEVERAGE	HEALTHY (YES OR NO)
	Breakfast	
	Snack	
	Lunch	
	Snack	
	Dinner	
	Other	

The Brain Warrior's Way Journal

DAY 9: DEVELOPING LASTING HABITS

Motivation Blast: Brain health is really easy: brain envy, avoid bad, do good.

What is my goal today?

_____

_____

_____

_____

Three things I am grateful for today

1. _____

2. _____

3. _____

Whom shall I appreciate today?

_____

_____

Today's Weight _____ Hours Slept _____

On a scale of 1 to 10 rate the following (1 = poor, 10 = great)

Mood ____ Energy ____ Focus ____
Memory ____ Inner peace ____ Decision making ____

Choose five brain healthy habits from the following list to do today

❑ Read my One Page Miracle

❑ Start the day with 16 to 20 ounces of water (8 to 10 ounces for kids)

- ❏ Focus on eating healthy without cheating
- ❏ Eat brain healthy snacks, maintain stable blood sugar
- ❏ Engage in smart exercise (bursting, weight training, coordination exercises)
- ❏ Learn something new
- ❏ Combat stress (hypnosis, meditation, brain-enhancing music)
- ❏ Learn from at least one mistake
- ❏ Get 7 to 8 hours of sleep
- ❏ Practice good decision making
- ❏ Take my supplements
- ❏ Connect with a Brain Warrior buddy
- ❏ Kill the ANTs

The Brain Warrior's Way Journal

DAY 9: BRAIN-ENHANCING FOOD

TIME	FOOD AND BEVERAGE	HEALTHY (YES OR NO)
	Breakfast	
	Snack	
	Lunch	
	Snack	
	Dinner	
	Other	

ARE CHEAT DAYS BLATANT SABOTAGE?

Do *not* schedule cheat days that trigger addiction and inflammation. Would therapists ever recommend cheat days for smokers, alcoholics, or sex addicts? Of course not. We've seen people eat as much as 4,000 calories of garbage with "self-permission," which is nonsense. Instead, choose *one* food that is not on your plan that day. And don't use the excuse that because you made one unhealthy choice, you might as well eat lousy for the entire day. How's that worked for you in the past? On average, it takes about three days to lose your cravings again after *only one day* of gorging on sugar and processed fat!

Always avoid your trigger foods. Be brutally honest with yourself about your addictions. If you know that you are still vulnerable to relapse, give yourself a couple more weeks, or even months, before loosening the reins. Tana had total control over food like pasta, burgers, fries, and even most sugary carbs after about two weeks. However, frosting was like crack for her and would have her in a dark corner of a doughnut shop, licking waxed paper for leftover traces—not pretty! She simply had to stay away from it for at least six months.

If you forget your healthful snack and find yourself hungry and faced with a smorgasbord of nonnutritious choices, make the healthiest selection possible from what's available. Ask yourself these questions: Is this healthy? Compared to what?

If you overindulge, make it a conscious decision. Lose the guilt, which serves only to cripple your progress. Then stop whining, be a warrior, and get back on track immediately. Think like your GPS, which doesn't call you a stupid idiot when you make a wrong turn. It just tells you to make the first legal U-turn.

Afterward, reflect on how it made you feel to choose food that you knew wasn't healthful. Turn bad days into good data. When we make a decision to eat food that doesn't serve us, we don't feel great, but being aware helps us be truthful and empowered. As a result we have very few of those days now . . . and we don't feel deprived for eating healthy.

The Brain Warrior's Way Journal

DAY 10: DEVELOPING LASTING HABITS

Motivation Blast: Who wants to be normal? Normal is unhealthy. Be optimal!

What is my goal today?

_____

_____

_____

_____

Three things I am grateful for today

1. _____

2. _____

3. _____

Whom shall I appreciate today?

_____

_____

Today's Weight _____ Hours Slept _____

On a scale of 1 to 10 rate the following (1 = poor, 10 = great)

Mood ____ Energy ____ Focus ____
Memory ____ Inner peace ____ Decision making ____

Choose five brain healthy habits from the following list to do today

❏ Read my One Page Miracle

❏ Start the day with 16 to 20 ounces of water (8 to 10 ounces for kids)

- ❏ Focus on eating healthy without cheating
- ❏ Eat brain healthy snacks, maintain stable blood sugar
- ❏ Engage in smart exercise (bursting, weight training, coordination exercises)
- ❏ Learn something new
- ❏ Combat stress (hypnosis, meditation, brain-enhancing music)
- ❏ Learn from at least one mistake
- ❏ Get 7 to 8 hours of sleep
- ❏ Practice good decision making
- ❏ Take my supplements
- ❏ Connect with a Brain Warrior buddy
- ❏ Kill the ANTs

The Brain Warrior's Way Journal

DAY 10: BRAIN-ENHANCING FOOD

TIME	FOOD AND BEVERAGE	HEALTHY (YES OR NO)
	Breakfast	
	Snack	
	Lunch	
	Snack	
	Dinner	
	Other	

TANA'S SLEEP, EXERCISE, AND FOOD ROUTINE

Sleep

Start with at least 8 hours of sleep, even when I travel; try to never take flights before 10:00 A.M. or after 3:00 P.M. so my sleep isn't affected. I go to bed early, often by 9:00.

Exercise

Work out with a trainer twice a week, lifting heavy weights and getting aerobic training.

Practice karate twice a week for high-intensity exercise and stretching.

Walk twice a week for more gentle recovery training.

Food (Try to Never Let Myself Get Hungry)

Start the day by hydrating with warm lemon and ginger water and a Pumpkin Spice-Up Cappuccino (see *The Brain Warrior's Way Cookbook*).

Breakfast

Breakfast smoothie *or* scrambled eggs with veggies

Snack

Chopped veggies with hummus or mashed avocados *or* ¼ cup nuts and a few berries

Lunch

Leftovers from night before *or* salad with protein, chili, or soup

Late-Afternoon Snack

Coconut wrap with almond butter or half an apple with almond butter and green tea

Dinner

Salad

Protein: fish, chicken, lamb, pork, or steak

Veggies: braised cauliflower, Brussels sprouts, or broccoli

Occasional sweet potato or quinoa

Dessert: one of my desserts on occasion (Luscious Lemon
   Squares or Two-Ingredient Nutty Butter Cups)

Fast for 12 hours from dinner to breakfast.

I eat this way 95 percent of the time. I rarely drink alcohol. Although I enjoy an occasional glass of wine, I know it doesn't love me back.

The Brain Warrior's Way Journal

DAY 11: DEVELOPING LASTING HABITS

Motivation Blast: Brain Warriors fight inflammation, oxidation, high blood sugar, nutrient depletion, and abnormal hormone levels. They fight the war on multiple fronts.

What is my goal today?

_____

_____

_____

_____

Three things I am grateful for today

1. _____

2. _____

3. _____

Whom shall I appreciate today?

_____

_____

Today's Weight _____ Hours Slept _____

On a scale of 1 to 10 rate the following (1 = poor, 10 = great)

Mood ____ Energy ____ Focus ____
Memory ____ Inner peace ____ Decision making ____

Choose five brain healthy habits from the following list to do today

❏ Read my One Page Miracle

❏ Start the day with 16 to 20 ounces of water (8 to 10 ounces for kids)

- ❏ Focus on eating healthy without cheating
- ❏ Eat brain healthy snacks, maintain stable blood sugar
- ❏ Engage in smart exercise (bursting, weight training, coordination exercises)
- ❏ Learn something new
- ❏ Combat stress (hypnosis, meditation, brain-enhancing music)
- ❏ Learn from at least one mistake
- ❏ Get 7 to 8 hours of sleep
- ❏ Practice good decision making
- ❏ Take my supplements
- ❏ Connect with a Brain Warrior buddy
- ❏ Kill the ANTs

The Brain Warrior's Way Journal

DAY 11: BRAIN-ENHANCING FOOD

TIME	FOOD AND BEVERAGE	HEALTHY (YES OR NO)
	Breakfast	
	Snack	
	Lunch	
	Snack	
	Dinner	
	Other	

The Brain Warrior's Way Journal

DAY 12: DEVELOPING LASTING HABITS

Motivation Blast: The best way to prevent accelerated aging and Alzheimer's disease is to prevent all the illnesses that are associated with them.

What is my goal today?

_____

_____

_____

_____

Three things I am grateful for today

1. _____

2. _____

3. _____

Whom shall I appreciate today?

_____

_____

Today's Weight _____ Hours Slept _____

On a scale of 1 to 10 rate the following (1 = poor, 10 = great)

Mood _____ Energy _____ Focus _____
Memory _____ Inner peace _____ Decision making _____

Choose five brain healthy habits from the following list to do today

❏ Read my One Page Miracle

❏ Start the day with 16 to 20 ounces of water (8 to 10 ounces for kids)

- Focus on eating healthy without cheating
- Eat brain healthy snacks, maintain stable blood sugar
- Engage in smart exercise (bursting, weight training, coordination exercises)
- Learn something new
- Combat stress (hypnosis, meditation, brain-enhancing music)
- Learn from at least one mistake
- Get 7 to 8 hours of sleep
- Practice good decision making
- Take my supplements
- Connect with a Brain Warrior buddy
- Kill the ANTs

The Brain Warrior's Way Journal

DAY 12: BRAIN-ENHANCING FOOD

TIME	FOOD AND BEVERAGE	HEALTHY (YES OR NO)
	Breakfast	
	Snack	
	Lunch	
	Snack	
	Dinner	
	Other	

LEARN FROM YOUR PAST SUCCESS

Using a past success as a template for overcoming bad habits is an excellent way to fuel future victory. Try picking a negative habit or pattern that you successfully overcame. Get clear about the wisdom you gleaned and lessons you learned and apply the *same strategy* to the current effort to change your unhealthy behaviors. The fact that you broke at least one bad habit is proof that you can do it again!

Consider the following questions as you meditate on a past success:

- At what point did I realize that I *had* to change?
- What was my leverage, my why?
- What had to happen in order for me to succeed?
- What were my beliefs about the challenge I faced?
- What steps were most productive as I worked toward my goal?
- How did I stay focused?
- How much effort and time did I invest in changing?
- Who offered me the most support? Who stood in my way?
- What techniques and skills served me best and which were ineffective?
- How did I feel when I broke the habit?

The Brain Warrior's Way Journal

DAY 13: DEVELOPING LASTING HABITS

Motivation Blast: Let every mistake you make be a valuable lesson.

What is my goal today?

_____

_____

_____

_____

Three things I am grateful for today

1. _____

2. _____

3. _____

Whom shall I appreciate today?

_____

_____

Today's Weight _____ Hours Slept _____

On a scale of 1 to 10 rate the following (1 = poor, 10 = great)

Mood ____ Energy ____ Focus ____
Memory ____ Inner peace ____ Decision making ____

Choose five brain healthy habits from the following list to do today

❏ Read my One Page Miracle

❏ Start the day with 16 to 20 ounces of water (8 to 10 ounces for kids)

- ❏ Focus on eating healthy without cheating
- ❏ Eat brain healthy snacks, maintain stable blood sugar
- ❏ Engage in smart exercise (bursting, weight training, coordination exercises)
- ❏ Learn something new
- ❏ Combat stress (hypnosis, meditation, brain-enhancing music)
- ❏ Learn from at least one mistake
- ❏ Get 7 to 8 hours of sleep
- ❏ Practice good decision making
- ❏ Take my supplements
- ❏ Connect with a Brain Warrior buddy
- ❏ Kill the ANTs

The Brain Warrior's Way Journal

DAY 13: BRAIN-ENHANCING FOOD

TIME	FOOD AND BEVERAGE	HEALTHY (YES OR NO)
	Breakfast	
	Snack	
	Lunch	
	Snack	
	Dinner	
	Other	

A NOTE ABOUT PLATEAUS

When you first start a health program and change your daily eating regimen, it's common to see rapid results in the first few weeks. However, your body eventually will adjust, and you may hit a plateau. This is very common with typical fad diets, but the Brain Warrior's Way takes your biology into account. We know that plateaus are often a normal process in a health program. We don't want you to equate plateaus with failure. Instead, use them as a gauge. Take an honest assessment of your progress and determine if you need to make adjustments. Here are some common reasons plateaus occur:

1. Initially, you may lose weight rapidly as a result of detoxification and decreasing inflammation. As you consume less toxic food and increase food that *detoxifies*, your body begins to release stored toxins. Eventually, it stabilizes and weight loss will take on a slower, steadier pace. Don't be discouraged—this is healthy!

2. Because fat cells store toxic material, your body needs time to clear the waste away. The plateau may be a signal that your body needs time to adjust to this shift. You can override this natural process and "diet" through it, but you will likely put your body under unnecessary stress and likely put the weight back on. Instead, try increasing your water intake, consuming more greens or green drinks, and participating in activities that cause you to sweat a little more, such as exercise and saunas. This process usually lasts for only a week or two.

3. It may be time to adjust your program and decrease your intake of animal protein a bit, replacing it with more wholesome choices. Once you lose a significant amount of weight, you will need to assess whether your food intake should be adjusted to your new size. A 220-pound person has different needs than a 180-pound person. You will still need to get regular doses of protein throughout the day, but possibly in smaller portions. Also, consider eating more vegetable sources of protein. Many people start to cut out one snack after they get cravings under control. Just don't

(CONTINUED)

go longer than 4 hours without something to keep your blood sugar stable and hormones balanced.

4. Go back to basics. What made you successful in the beginning when you were zealous about following the program closely? Many people unwittingly slip back into old habits if not kept in check. Those two bites of your kid's pancakes add up, along with the forgotten popcorn over the weekend. . . . You get the idea. When you hit a plateau, it's time to journal, start measuring, and write down everything you eat for a couple of weeks. A couple of extra bites here and there can really add up.

5. Review your exercise program. Sometimes a weight-loss plateau coincides with an exercise plateau—it may be time to push your workouts up a notch. Increasing muscle mass is a great way to rev your metabolism without drastically cutting calories.

6. Turn to your tribe for support. Having a coach, mentor, or friend for support and accountability can make all the difference. People who participate in health programs together double their weight loss and report sticking with their program.

The Brain Warrior's Way Journal

DAY 14: DEVELOPING LASTING HABITS

Motivation Blast: It's not about you. It is about generations of you.

What is my goal today?

_____

_____

_____

_____

Three things I am grateful for today

1. _____

2. _____

3. _____

Whom shall I appreciate today?

_____

_____

Today's Weight _____ Hours Slept _____

On a scale of 1 to 10 rate the following (1 = poor, 10 = great)

Mood ____ Energy ____ Focus ____
Memory ____ Inner peace ____ Decision making ____

Choose five brain healthy habits from the following list to do today

❏ Read my One Page Miracle

❏ Start the day with 16 to 20 ounces of water (8 to 10 ounces for kids)

- ❏ Focus on eating healthy without cheating
- ❏ Eat brain healthy snacks, maintain stable blood sugar
- ❏ Engage in smart exercise (bursting, weight training, coordination exercises)
- ❏ Learn something new
- ❏ Combat stress (hypnosis, meditation, brain-enhancing music)
- ❏ Learn from at least one mistake
- ❏ Get 7 to 8 hours of sleep
- ❏ Practice good decision making
- ❏ Take my supplements
- ❏ Connect with a Brain Warrior buddy
- ❏ Kill the ANTs

The Brain Warrior's Way Journal

DAY 14: BRAIN-ENHANCING FOOD

TIME	FOOD AND BEVERAGE	HEALTHY (YES OR NO)
Breakfast		
Snack		
Lunch		
Snack		
Dinner		
Other		

WHEN YOU CHANGE, OTHERS ARE LIKELY TO FOLLOW—ALTHOUGH PERHAPS NOT RIGHT AWAY

Once you start doing the right things for yourself and those you love, your world will start to change, but maybe not instantly. Patience is often required.

While Daniel was growing up, his father, Lou, was not always easy on him, and Daniel was not always easy for his dad. Lou is a very successful, driven, blunt man whose first favorite word is *bullshit* and second favorite word is *no*. Like many successful entrepreneurs, he tells it like he sees it. He owns a chain of grocery stores in Southern California and was a long-term chairman of the board of Unified Grocers, a $4 billion company.

In 1980, when Daniel told his dad he was going to be a psychiatrist, Lou got mad at him. "Why don't you want to be a real doctor? Why do you want to be a nut doctor and hang out with nuts all day long?" To say Lou was not psychologically minded would be an understatement.

Lou also had a blind spot when it came to his own health. He thought he was invincible. "I give heart attacks," he told people repeatedly over the years. "I don't get them." When Daniel encouraged his dad to get healthy, Lou belittled him and called him a health nut. And so it went, until one day Lou was sick of being sick.

At age eighty-three, Lou developed atrial fibrillation, a heart arrhythmia, which made him feel extremely tired, dizzy, and short of breath. He underwent a heart procedure (cardioversion) and resumed a normal heart rhythm for two years. We felt like he dodged a bullet. Then two years later, mold was discovered in his home and he had to move out for four months. During that time he developed a horrible cough and the abnormal heart rhythm returned. He was tired and short of breath, couldn't sleep, had to stop driving, and stopped going to work, which had been his passion for the last sixty-five years. This time none of the medical treatments worked, including three more cardioversions and multiple medications—and he felt terrible for months. His blood sugar was high, and he had very high levels of inflammation.

Then one day, when Daniel was at his home, his father, looking so sad, said, "Danny, what do you want me to do? I can't take this anymore. I am so sick of being sick."

"Dad, I need you to just do everything I am going to tell you to do," Daniel pleaded. "I promise it won't be hard. Don't cheat and be diligent for just a few weeks."

Lou's stubborn personality kicked in the way we have seen with many men when they finally make the decision to get serious about changing. He did everything we asked him to do, especially getting his diet right. We told him there was no room for error. He would text us ingredient labels and ask us if he could eat this or that. He had owned grocery stores for more than sixty years, but when he developed an awareness of healthy and unhealthy foods, he was dismayed by the vast amount of awful food he sold in his stores and had put in his body.

Once he emotionally bought into the Brain Warrior's Way, he was all in. Over the next six months Lou lost thirty-five pounds; he and Daniel started working out together, lifting weights. Over time, he was able to do planks for three minutes at a time (see the photo below). His energy improved and, at the time of this writing, he is feeling better than he has in years. Our promise to him was that he could be feeling better at ninety than he did at seventy by making the right decisions and engaging in the right habits.

BRAIN WARRIORS LOU AND DANIEL

Lou then started talking about Daniel in a new way to his six other children. The "health nut" and "nut doctor" days were finally gone, and Lou would often say, "Your brother wouldn't like you eating that. . . .

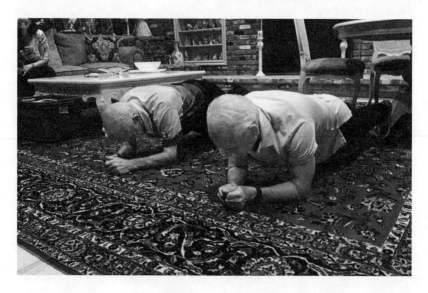

You could be making better choices. . . . What would your brother say about that decision?" Daniel's siblings were tired of hearing "Daniel this" and "Daniel that." But for Daniel, it made all the years of belittlement worth the pain.

In a vulnerable moment Daniel's father said, "I never thought it would ever happen to me." Aging and death are coming for all of us. We can encourage them to come early or we can discourage them, because we believe our lives matter and there is a purpose for us on the planet. We choose to discourage disease and death, as Lou is doing now. It is never too late to be a health nut, but don't wait until you are sick of being sick. The only reason Lou got well was because we modeled the message and persisted living the Brain Warrior's Way, despite being belittled and criticized. By choosing this path and being patient—sometimes for decades—you may be able to make a radical difference in yourself and those you love.

Brain Warrior
Dos and Don'ts

■

BRAIN WARRIOR DOS

- Make great decisions—it changes everything.
- Have a sheepdog mind-set.
- Define and focus on your purpose.
- Identify with being strong, serious, and healthy.
- Be a good parent to yourself: firm and kind.
- Focus on abundance, never deprivation: Focus on an abundance of amazing habits to deprive yourself of a lifetime of illness and aging.
- Be an accurate, honest, cautiously optimistic thinker.
- Have appropriate anxiety.
- Be aware of the mass propaganda weapons and psychological warfare.
- Be aware that trouble potentially lurks in hospitals, doctors' offices, schools, business, and churches.
- Have a clear strategy: Brain envy means avoiding bad and doing good.
- Assess your brain.
- Know your brain type.
- Optimize your important numbers—don't just normalize them.
- Fight the war on multiple fronts (blood flow, inflammation, gut health, blood sugar stabilization, healthy acetylcholine, serotonin and dopamine levels, antioxidant support, nerve cell membrane fluidity, and nutrient loading).

- Always engage in prevention strategies.
- Protect your brain.
- Be on a cancer prevention program.
- Get mental health issues treated (ADD/ADHD, depression, PTSD, anxiety disorders, bipolar disorder, etc.).
- Breathe clean air.
- Engage in smart exercise.
- Create social support.
- Maintain a healthy weight.
- Manage stress.
- Sleep 7 to 8 hours.
- Take basic and targeted supplements.
- Meditate.
- Use light therapy, if needed.
- Do neurofeedback.
- Have loving relationships.
- Eat according to Brain Warrior nutrition guidelines.
  - Think high-quality calories and not too many of them. Calories matter, but quality matters more.
  - Drink plenty of water and don't drink too many of your calories.
  - Eat high-quality protein in small doses throughout the day.
  - Eat smart carbohydrates (low glycemic, high fiber).
  - Focus your diet on healthy fats.
  - Eat from the rainbow, which means healthy foods of many different colors (not Skittles).
  - Cook with brain healthy herbs and spices to boost your brain and body.
  - Make sure your food is as clean as possible: organic, hormone free, antibiotic free, grass fed, and free range.
  - If you struggle with any mental health or physical issue, eliminate any potential allergens or internal attackers, such as MSG, gluten, corn, soy, and dairy.
  - Read the labels.
- Start each day with intention, gratitude and appreciation.
- Practice accelerated mindfulness.
  - Slow your breathing when exhaling.
  - Kill the ANTs.

- ▶ Self-hypnosis.
- ▶ Heart rate variability.
- ▶ Loving-kindness meditation.
- ▶ Brain-enhancement playlist.
- ▶ Be curious, not furious and learn from each mistake.
- Turn your pain into purpose.
- Know what you would die for.
- Ask yourself, "Why is the world a better place because I breathe?"
- Be serious, relentless, and responsible as a Brain Warrior.
- Know that the right social connections make you smarter; the wrong ones hurt you.
- Be careful with whom you spend time.
- Spend time with healthy people.
- Once you know this information, it's your responsibility to act on it for the benefit of those you love.
- Have a sense of urgency—now is the time to act.
- Spend at least a year putting these habits into your life.
- Understand the timing of primitive, mechanical, and spontaneous phases.
- Engage in the 14-Day Brain Boost.
- Clean out your pantry.

BRAIN WARRIOR DON'TS

- Make bad decisions.
- Focus on short-term pain versus long-term pain.
- Engage in risky behavior.
- Get little to no physical activity.
- Stop learning.
- Smoke.
- Use marijuana, cocaine, methamphetamine, LSD, or other mind-altering drugs.
- Have low blood sugar levels.
- Have high blood sugar levels.
- Develop diabetes or prediabetes.
- Develop hypertension or prehypertension.
- Be obese.
- Think "everything in moderation."

- Avoid getting sleep apnea treatment.
- Ingest artificial food dyes and additives.
- Expose yourself to air and water pollution.
- Expose yourself to environmental toxins.
- Risk oxygen deprivation.
- Have vitamin or hormone deficiencies.
- Be frail.
- Ignore insomnia.

LIMIT

- Gadgets.
- Chronic stress.
- General anesthesia.
- Alcohol.
- Caffeine.
- Sugar.
- Gluten (unless sensitive, then eliminate it).
- Corn.
- Soy.
- Dairy.
- Time with unhealthy family and friends.

About the Authors

■

DANIEL G. AMEN, MD

Daniel Amen believes that brain health is central to all health and success. When your brain works right, he says, you work right; and when your brain is troubled you are much more likely to have trouble in your life. His work is dedicated to helping people have better brains and better lives.

The Washington Post wrote that Dr. Amen is the most popular psychiatrist in America and Sharecare named him the Web's number one most influential expert on and advocate for mental health.

Dr. Amen is a physician, double board-certified psychiatrist, and ten-time *New York Times* bestselling author. He is the founder of Amen Clinics in Costa Mesa and Walnut Creek, California; Bellevue, Washington; Reston, Virginia; Atlanta, Georgia; and New York City. Amen Clinics have the world's largest database of functional brain scans relating to behavior, totaling more than 125,000 scans on patients from 111 countries.

Dr. Amen is a Distinguished Fellow of the American Psychiatric Association, the highest award given to members, and is the lead researcher on the world's largest brain imaging and rehabilitation study on professional football players. His research has not only demonstrated high levels of brain damage in players but also shown the possibility of significant recovery for many with the principles that underlie his work.

Together with Pastor Rick Warren and Dr. Mark Hyman, Dr. Amen is also one of the chief architects of Saddleback Church's "Daniel Plan," a program to get the world healthy through religious organizations.

Dr. Amen has written, produced and hosted eleven popular shows about the brain, which have aired more than 100,000 times across North America.

Dr. Amen is the author or coauthor of more than seventy-five professional articles, seven book chapters, and over 30 books, including the number one *New York Times* bestsellers *The Daniel Plan; Change Your Brain, Change Your Life*; *Magnificent Mind at Any Age; Change Your Brain, Change Your Body; Use Your Brain to Change Your Age; Unleash the Power of the Female Brain*; and *Healing ADD*.

Dr. Amen's published scientific articles have appeared in the prestigious journals *Brain Imaging and Behavior, Journal of Alzheimer's Disease, Molecular Psychiatry, PLoS ONE*, Nature's *Translational Psychiatry, Nature Obesity, Journal of Neuropsychiatry and Clinical Neuroscience*, and *Journal of Neurotrauma*, among others. His research on post-traumatic stress disorder and traumatic brain injury was recognized by *Discover* magazine as one of the top 100 stories in science in 2015.

Dr. Amen has appeared in movies, including *After the Last Round* and *The Crash Reel*, and has appeared in Emmy-winning shows, such as *The Truth About Drinking* and the *Dr. Oz Show*. He was a consultant on the movie *Concussion*. He has also spoken for the National Security Agency (NSA), the National Science Foundation (NSF), Harvard's Learning and the Brain Conference, the Department of the Interior, the National Council of Juvenile and Family Court Judges, and the Supreme Courts of Delaware, Ohio, and Wyoming. Dr. Amen's work has been featured in *Newsweek, Time,* Huffington Post, *ABC World News, 20/20,* BBC, London *Telegraph, Parade Magazine, New York Times, New York Times Magazine, Washington Post, LA Times, Men's Health*, and *Cosmopolitan*.

Dr. Amen is married to Tana, the father of four children, and grandfather to Elias, Emmy, Liam, and Louie. He is an avid table tennis player.

TANA AMEN, RN, BSN

Tana Amen helps people realize that they are not stuck with the brain and body they have by empowering them with simple strategies that will transform them into *warriors* for their health. Tana is the executive vice president of Amen Clinics, *New York Times* bestselling author of *The Omni Diet*, a highly respected health and fitness expert, and a nationally renowned speaker and media guest.

Tana and Daniel have written and hosted together three national public television shows: *Healing ADD, The Omni Health Revolution*, and *The Brain Warrior's Way*. Working side by side, they are creating an army of people dedicated to transforming the health of their brains and bodies using the tips and strategies in the Brain Warrior's Way.

In addition to being a guest on *The Doctors, The Today Show, Good Day New York, Extra, Joy Behar,* and other shows, Tana has given presentations at the American Academy of Anti-Aging Medicine, Saddleback Church, High Performance Academy, Superhero You, the Institute for the Advancement of Human Behavior, the Omega Institute, Kripalu, Beacon House, Salvation Army Adult Rehabilitation Center, and many other wellness-focused organizations.

After graduating Magna Cum Laude from Loma Linda University's School of Nursing, Tana spent years working at Loma Linda's level A trauma unit as a neurosurgical intensive care nurse, taking care of some of the sickest patients in the hospital. There she learned firsthand the value of diet and nutrition on brain health. Tana is the author of six highly successful books, including *The Omni Diet, Healing ADD Through Food, Change Your Brain, Change Your Body Cookbook, Get Healthy with the Brain Doctor's Wife, Eat Healthy with the Brain Doctor's Wife*, and *Live Longer with the Brain Doctor's Wife*.

In addition to working with her husband at Amen Clinics, Tana was a nutrition consultant and coach as well as being part of the team that included psychiatrist Dr. Daniel Amen, functional medicine specialist Dr. Mark Hyman, and heart surgeon Dr. Mehmet Oz that helped create the wildly popular Daniel Plan (danielplan.com) for Saddleback Church at the request of Pastor Rick Warren.

Tana hosts a unique tribe of Brain Warriors at the Amens' community, Brain Fit Life (mybrainfitlife.com), where she shares healthy eating tips and lifestyle strategies. She has also played an important part in Dr. Amen's successful PBS specials.

Tana practices martial arts regularly and has a black belt in Kenpo and Tae Kwan Do. Being a mother and wife is Tana's first passion. Keeping her family and friends focused on fitness and health is a primary value for her. Tana believes that *everyone* can optimize his or her health by using the Brain Warrior's Way.

Gratitude and Appreciation

■

So many people have been involved in the process of creating this book and helping us create brain health warriors. We are grateful for and appreciate the following:

The tens of thousands of patients and families who have believed in our work and allowed the staff at Amen Clinics and us to help them have better brains and better lives.

Dr. David Ludwig, who read the book and gave us very helpful scientific and editorial feedback.

The amazing staff and physicians at Amen Clinics. As we write this, we currently serve 4,000 patient visits a month, making us one of the most active private mental and brain health centers in the world. Our professionals work hard every day serving our patients. Special appreciation to our fearless leader, CEO Terry Weber, and colleagues Tiffany Lesko and Jenny Faherty, who read every word of this book to make sure they made sense and were easy to understand, as well as Tana's brand leader, Jasmine Patterson, who is a constant source of energy and creativity. We are also grateful to our creative director, C. J. Ramos, who was instrumental in the cover design.

Our professional colleagues who believed in us and sent us their patients for evaluation through the years.

Bob and Barbara White, our Kenpo instructors, who have taught us many valuable lessons.

Our original editor at Penguin, Denise Silvestro, who believed in this book and helped make it possible as well as others at Penguin, including Allison Janice, Tom Colgan, Jin Yu, and Claire Zion.

Our friends and colleagues at public television stations across the country, including mentors and friends Alan Foster, Alicia Steele, Kurt Mendelsohn, BaBette Davidson, Greg Sherwood, Camille Dixon, Stacey Wiggins, and Maura Phinney. Public television is a treasure and we are grateful to be able to partner with stations to bring our message of hope and healing to millions.

Our family, who has lived through our obsession with everything Brain Warrior's Way, especially our children Antony, Breanne, Kaitlyn, and Chloe, our grandchildren, and our parents, Mary Meeks (Tana's mom) and Louis and Dorie Amen. We know that many times you were tired of listening about the brain, but nonetheless gave us unending support.

Resources

∎

AMEN CLINICS, INC.

amenclinics.com

Amen Clinics, Inc. (ACI) was established in 1989 by Daniel G. Amen, MD. We specialize in innovative diagnosis and treatment planning for a wide variety of behavioral, learning, emotional, cognitive, and weight issues for children, teenagers, and adults. ACI has an international reputation for evaluating brain-behavior problems, such as ADD, depression, anxiety, school failure, traumatic brain injury and concussions, obsessive-compulsive disorders, aggressiveness, marital conflict, cognitive decline, brain toxicity from drugs or alcohol, and obesity. In addition, we work with people to optimize brain function and decrease the risk for Alzheimer's disease and other age-related issues.

Brain SPECT imaging is performed in the clinics. ACI has the world's largest database of brain scans for emotional, cognitive, and behavioral problems. ACI welcomes referrals from physicians, psychologists, social workers, marriage and family therapists, drug and alcohol counselors, and individual patients and families.

Our toll-free number is 888-564-2700.

Amen Clinics Orange County, California
3150 Bristol St., Suite 400
Costa Mesa, CA 92626

Amen Clinics San Francisco Bay Area
350 Wiget Lane, Suite 100
Walnut Creek, CA 94598

Amen Clinics Northwest
616 120th Ave. NE, Suite C100
Bellevue, WA 98005

Amen Clinics Washington, DC
10701 Parkridge Blvd., Suite 110
Reston, VA 20191

Amen Clinics New York
16 East 40th St., 9th Floor
New York, NY 10016
(888) 564-2700

Amen Clinics Atlanta
5901-C Peachtree Dunwoody Road, N.E., Suite 65
Atlanta, GA 30328
(888) 564-2700

The Amen Clinics website (amenclinics.com) is an educational, interactive site geared toward mental health and medical professionals, educators, students, and the general public. It contains a wealth of information and resources to help you learn about optimizing your brain. The site contains more than 300 color brain SPECT images, thousands of scientific abstracts on brain SPECT imaging for psychiatry, a free brain health assessment, and much, much more.

BRAIN FIT LIFE

mybrainfitlife.com

Based on Dr. Amen's thirty-five years as a clinical psychiatrist, this sophisticated online community was developed by Dr. Amen and his wife, Tana, to help you feel smarter, happier, and younger. It includes

- Detailed questionnaires to help you know your brain type and a personalized program targeted to your own needs
- WebNeuro, a sophisticated neuropsychological test to assess your brain

- Fun brain games and tools to boost your motivation
- Exclusive, award-winning, 24/7 brain gym membership
- Physical exercises and tutorials led by Tana
- Hundreds of Tana's delicious brain healthy recipes
- Exercises to kill the ANTs
- Meditation and hypnosis audios for sleep, anxiety, overcoming weight issues, pain, and peak performance
- Amazing brain-enhancing music from Grammy Award winner Barry Goldstein
- Online forum for questions and answers and a community of support
- Access to monthly live coaching calls with Daniel and Tana

BRAINMD HEALTH

brainmdhealth.com

For the highest-quality brain health supplements, courses, books, and information products.

Endnotes

∎

INTRODUCTION: THE BRAIN WARRIOR'S WAY

1   Panel on Understanding Cross-National Health Differences Among High-Income Countries, *U.S. Health in International Perspective: Shorter Lives, Poorer Health* (Washington, DC: National Academy of Sciences, Institute of Medicine, 2013).

2   "Kids Meals, Toys, and TV Advertising: A Triple Threat to Child Health," *Journal of Pediatrics,* October 30, 2015, available at www.jpeds.com/content/JPEDSEmond.

3   A. L. Howard, M. Robinson, G. J. Smith, et al., "ADHD Is Associated with a 'Western' Dietary Pattern in Adolescents," *Journal of Attention Disorders* 15, no. 5 (2011): 403–11; F. N. Jacka, N. Cherbuin, K. J. Anstey, and P. Butterworth, "Dietary Patterns and Depressive Symptoms over Time: Examining the Relationships with Socioeconomic Position, Health Behaviours and Cardiovascular Risk," *PLoS ONE* 9, no. 1 (2014): e87657; B. Shakersain, G. Santoni, S. C. Larsson, et al., "Prudent Diet May Attenuate the Adverse Effects of Western Diet on Cognitive Decline. *Alzheimer's & Dementia: Journal of the Alzheimer's Association* 12, no. 2 (2016): 100–9; and G. Tarantino, V. Citro, and C. Finelli, "Hype or Reality: Should Patients with Metabolic Syndrome-Related NAFLD Be on the Hunter-Gatherer (Paleo) Diet to Decrease Morbidity?," *Journal of Gastrointestinal and Liver Diseases* 24, no. 3 (2015): 359–68.

4   F. N. Jacka, N. Cherbuin, K. J. Anstey, et al., "Western Diet Is Associated with a Smaller Hippocampus: A Longitudinal Investigation," *BMC Medicine* 13 (2015): 215.

5   N. Singer, "Can't Put Down Your Device? That's by Design," *New York Times,* December 5, 2015.

6   V. Rideout, *Common Sense Census: Media Use by Tweens and Teens* (San Francisco: Common Sense, 2015).

7   J. B. Weaver 3rd, D. Mays, S. Sargent Weaver, et al., "Health-Risk Correlates of Video-Game Playing among Adults," *American Journal of Preventive Medicine* 37, no. 4 (2009): 299–305.

8   N. E. R. Hoover, *Hooked: How to Build Habit-Forming Products* (New York: Penguin Group USA, 2014).

9   K. McSpadden, "You Now Have a Shorter Attention Span Than a Goldfish," *Time,* May 14, 2015.

10 H. Bruch and S. Ghoshal, "Beware the Busy Manager," *Harvard Business Review* 80, no. 2 (2002): 62–69.

11 H. Chui, D. Gerstorf, C. A. Hoppmann, and M. A. Luszcz, "Trajectories of Depressive Symptoms in Old Age: Integrating Age-, Pathology-, and Mortality-Related Changes," *Psychology and Aging* 30, no. 4 (2015): 940–51.

12 A. S. S. Cohen, "ADHD Seen in 11% of U.S. Children as Diagnoses Rise," *New York Times,* April 1, 2013.

13 A. Menke, S. Casagrande, L. Geiss, and C. C. Cowie, "Prevalence of and Trends in Diabetes among Adults in the United States, 1988–2012," *Journal of the American Medical Association* 314, no. 10 (2015): 1021–29.

14 M. Hyman, *Eat Fat, Get Thin: Why the Fat We Eat Is the Key to Sustained Weight Loss and Vibrant Health* (New York: Little, Brown, 2016).

15   J. Holt-Lunstad, T. B. Smith, M. Baker, et al. "Loneliness and Social Isolation as Risk Factors for Mortality: A Meta-Analytic Review," *Perspectives on Psychological Science* 10, no. 2 (2015): 227–37.

16   A. Heguy, "How Do Herding Dogs Drive Away Wolves and Protect Flocks of Sheep When We Know Wolves Are Stronger Than Dogs?" Quora, June 28, 2015, available at quora.com/How-do-herding-dogs-drive-away-wolves-and-protect-flocks-of-sheep-when-we-know-wolves-are-stronger-than-dogs.

17   S. Schoenian, "Sheep Behavior," Sheep 201: A Beginner's Guide to Raising Sheep, last updated June 18, 2011, available at sheep101.info/201/behavior.html.

18   T. A. Press, "450 Sheep Jump to Their Deaths in Turkey," *USA Today* online, July 8, 2005. http://usatoday30.usatoday.com/news/offbeat/2005-07-08-sheep-suicide_x.htm.

19   Edisonone, "Xinjiang Sheep Herd Jumps to Their Deaths off Cliff," China Daily Forum, June 5, 2014, available at blog.chinadaily.com.cn/thread-980751-1-1.html.

20   R. B. Cohen, C. Bavishi, and A. Rozanski, "Purpose in Life and Its Relationship to All-Cause Mortality and Cardiovascular Events: A Meta-Analysis," paper presented at the Epi Lifestyle 2015 Scientific Sessions meeting of the American Heart Association, March 3–4, 2015, Baltimore, MD; and P. L. Hill and N. A. Turiano, "Purpose in Life as a Predictor of Mortality across Adulthood," *Psychological Science* 25, no. 7 (2014): 1482–86.

21   M. C. Otto, N. S. Padhye, A. G. Bertoni, et al., "Everything in Moderation—Dietary Diversity and Quality, Central Obesity and Risk of Diabetes," *PloS ONE* 10, no. 10 (2015): e0141341.

22   M. Rao, A. Afshin, G. Singh, and D. Mozaffarian, "Do Healthier Foods and Diet Patterns Cost More Than Less Healthy Options? A systematic Review and Meta-Analysis," *BMJ Open* 3, no. 12 (2013): e004277.

PART 2: ASSESSMENT OF A BRAIN WARRIOR

23   H. Friedman and L. Martin, *The Longevity Project: Surprising Discoveries for Health and Long Life from the Landmark Eight-Decade Study* (New York: Plume, 2012).

24   B. M. Kuehn, "The Brain Fights Back: New Approaches to Mitigating Cognitive Decline," *Journal of the American Medical Association* 314, no. 23 (2015): 2492–94.

25   K. B. Rajan, R. S. Wilson, J. Weuve, et al., "Cognitive Impairment 18 Years before Clinical Diagnosis of Alzheimer Disease Dementia," *Neurology* 85, no. 10 (2015): 898–904.

26   A. J. Kiliaan, I. A. Arnoldussen, and D. R. Gustafson, "Adipokines: A Link between Obesity and Dementia?" *Lancet Neurology* 13, no. 9 (2014): 913–23; and S. Garcia-Ptacek, G. Faxen-Irving, P. Cermakova, et al., "Body Mass Index in Dementia," *European Journal of Clinical Nutrition* 68, no. 11 (2014): 1204–9.

27   K. Deckers, M. P. van Boxtel, O. J. Schiepers, et al., "Target Risk Factors for Dementia Prevention: A Systematic Review and Delphi Consensus Study on the Evidence from Observational Studies," *International Journal of Geriatric Psychiatry* 30, no.3 (2015): (201s):234–46. doi: 10.1002/gps.4245. Epub 2014 Dec 12.

28   C. R. Pacanowski and D. A. Levitsky, "Frequent Self-Weighing and Visual Feedback for Weight Loss in Overweight Adults," *Journal of Obesity*, June 2015, Article ID 763680, 9 pages, doi:10.1155/2015/763680.

29   I. Hajjar, V. Marmerelis, D. C. Shin, and H. Chui, "Assessment of Cerebrovascular Reactivity during Resting State Breathing and Its Correlation with Cognitive Function in Hypertension," *Cerebrovascular Diseases* 38, no. 1 (2014): 10–16.

30   CDC, "High Blood Pressure Facts 2015," last updated February 19, 2015, available at cdc.gov/bloodpressure/facts.htm.

31   C. A. Peterson, A. K. Tosh, and A. M. Belenchia, "Vitamin D Insufficiency and Insulin Resistance in Obese Adolescents," *Therapeutic Advances in Endocrinology and Metabolism* 5, no. 6 (2014): 166–89.

32   M. A. Polak, L. A. Houghton, A. I. Reeder, et al., "Serum 25-Hydroxyvitamin D Concentrations and Depressive Symptoms among Young Adult Men and Women, *Nutrients* 6, no. 11 (2014): 4720–30.

33   L. Perna, U. Mons, M. Kliegel, and H. Brenner, "Serum 25-Hydroxyvitamin D and Cognitive Decline: A Longitudinal Study among Nondemented Older Adults," *Dementia and Geriatric Cognitive Disorders* 38, nos. 3–4 (2014): 254–63; and M. Schlogl and M. F. Holick, "Vitamin D and Neurocognitive Function," *Clinical Interventions in Aging* 9 (2014): 559–68.

34   T. Ruwanpathirana, C. M. Reid, A. J. Owen, et al., "Assessment of Vitamin D and Its Association with Cardiovascular Disease Risk Factors in an Adult Migrant Population: An Audit of Patient Records at a Community Health Centre in Kensington, Melbourne, Australia," *BMC Cardiovascular Disorders* 14 (2014): 157; and S. Khadanga and C. V. Massey, "Incidence of Vitamin D Insufficiency in Coastal South-Eastern US Patient Population with Cardiovascular Disease," *Journal of Clinical Medicine Research* 6, no. 6 (2014): 469–75.

35   M. Hewison, "An Update on Vitamin D and Human Immunity," Clinical Endocrinology 76, no. 3 (2012): 315–25; and T. Sahay and A. N. Ananthakrishnan, "Vitamin D Deficiency Is Associated with Community-Acquired Clostridium Difficile Infection: A Case-Control Study," *BMC Infectious Diseases* 14 (2014): 661.

36   J. Wranicz and D. Szostak-Wegierek, "Health Outcomes of Vitamin D. Part II. Role in Prevention of Diseases" *Roczniki Panstwowego Zakladu Higieny* 65, no. 4 (2014): 273–79.

37   M. Belvederi Murri, M. Respino, M. Masotti, et al., "Vitamin D and Psychosis: Mini Meta-Analysis," *Schizophrenia Research* 150, no. 1 (2013): 235–39.

38   S. Afzal, P. Brondum-Jacobsen, S. E. Bojesen, and B. G. Nordestgaard, "Genetically Low Vitamin D Concentrations and Increased Mortality: Mendelian Randomisation Analysis in Three Large Cohorts," *British Medical Journal* 349 (2014): g6330; and G. Bjelakovic, L. L. Gluud, D. Nikolova, et al., "Vitamin D Supplementation for Prevention of Mortality in Adults," *Cochrane Database of Systematic Reviews* 1 (2014): 007470.

39   A. C. Nowakowski, "Chronic Inflammation and Quality of Life in Older Adults: A Cross-Sectional Study Using Biomarkers to Predict Emotional and Relational Outcomes," *Health and Quality of Life Outcomes* 12 (2014): 141; doi: 10.1186/s12955-014-0141-0. M. G. O'Doherty, T. Jorgensen, A. Borglykke, et al., "Repeated Measures of Body Mass Index and C-Reactive Protein in Relation to All-Cause Mortality and Cardiovascular Disease: Results from the Consortium on Health and Ageing Network of Cohorts in Europe and the United States (CHANCES)," *European Journal of Epidemiology* Dec 29 (12) (2014): 887–97; and J. M. Chen, G. H. Cui, G. X. Jiang, et al., "Cognitive Impairment among Elderly Individuals in Shanghai Suburb, China: Association of C-Reactive Protein and Its Interactions with Other Relevant Factors," *American Journal of Alzheimer's Disease and Other Dementias* 29, no. 8 (2014): 712–17.

40   D. G. Amen, J. C. Wu, D. Taylor, and K Willeumier, "Reversing Brain Damage in Former NFL Players: Implications for Traumatic Brain Injury and Substance Abuse Rehabilitation," *Journal of Psychoactive Drugs* 43, no. 1 (2011): 1–5.

41   K. A. Tsvetanov, R. N. Henson, L. K. Tyler, et al., "The Effect of Ageing on fMRI: Correction for the Confounding Effects of Vascular Reactivity Evaluated by Joint fMRI and MEG in 335 Adults," *Human Brain Mapping* 36, no. 6 (2015): 48–69; doi: 10.1002/hbm.22768.

42   H. A. Feldman, I. Goldstein, D. G. Hatzichristou, et al., "Impotence and Its Medical and Psychosocial Correlates: Results of the Massachusetts Male Aging Study," *Journal of Urology* 151, no. 1 (1994): 54–61.

43   A. C. Logan and M. Katzman "Major Depressive Disorder: Probiotics May Be an Adjuvant Therapy," *Medical Hypotheses* 64, no. 3 (2005): 533–38.

44   W. Xu, L. Tan, H. F. Wan, et al., "Meta-Analysis of Modifiable Risk Factors for Alzheimer's Disease," *Journal of Neurology, Neurosurgery, and Psychiatry* 86, no. 12 (2015): 1299–1306.

45   C. C. Chung, D. Pimentel, A. J. Jor'dan, et al., "Inflammation-Associated Declines in Cerebral Vasoreactivity and Cognition in Type 2 Diabetes," *Neurology* 85, no. 5 (2015): 450–58.

46   I. Efimova, N. Efimova, and Y. Lishmanov, "Cerebral Blood Flow and Cognitive Function in Patients with Metabolic Syndrome: Effect of Antihypertensive Therapy," *Journal of Clinical Hypertension* 16, no. 12 (2014): 900–6.

47   S. Knapton, "Type 2 Diabetes Can Be Cured through Weight Loss, Newcastle University Finds," *Telegraph*, May 14, 2016.

48   D. S. Hasin, T. D. Saha, B. T. Kerridge, et al., "Prevalence of Marijuana Use Disorders in the United States between 2001–2002 and 2012–2013," *JAMA Psychiatry* 72, no. 12 (2015): 1235–42.

49   A. G. Amen and M. Waugh, "High Resolution Brain SPECT Imaging of Marijuana Smokers with AD/HD," *Journal of Psychoactive Drugs* 30, no. 2 (1998): 209–14.

50   K. Abernathy, L. J. Chandler, and J. J. Woodward, "Alcohol and the Prefrontal Cortex," *International Review of Neurobiology* 91 (2010): 289–320.

51   R. Tikkanen, J. Tiihonen, M. R. Rautiainen, et al., "Impulsive Alcohol-Related Risk-Behavior and Emotional Dysregulation among Individuals with a Serotonin 2B Receptor Stop Codon," *Translational Psychiatry* 5 (2015): 681.

52   R. P. Winograd, D. L. Steinley, and D. J. Sher, "Drunk Personality: Reports from Drinkers and Knowledgeable Informants," *Experimental and Clinical Psychopharmacology* 22, no. 3 (2014): 187–97.

53   A. Smyth, K. K. Teo, S. Rangarajan, et al., "Alcohol Consumption and Cardiovascular Disease, Cancer, Injury, Admission to Hospital, and Mortality: A Prospective Cohort Study," *Lancet* 386, no. 10007 (2015): 1945–54.

54   D. Praud, M. Rota, J. Rehm, et al., "Cancer Incidence and Mortality Attributable to Alcohol Consumption," *International Journal of Cancer* 138, no. 6 (2016): 1380–87.

55   J. K. S. Rehm, *Alcohol Consumption* (Lyon, France: International Agency for Research on Cancer, 2014).

56   S. Borland, "Month Off Drinking Slashes Risk of Disease: Abstaining Found to Heal the Liver and Lower Blood Pressure and Cholesterol Levels," DailyMail.com, October 25, 2015.

57   M. J. Cordi, A. A. Schlarb, and B. Rasch, "Deepening Sleep by Hypnotic Suggestion," *Sleep* 37, no. 6 (2014): 1143–52, 52A–52F.

58   C. Gulli, "A Newfound Link between Brain Injuries and ADHD," Macleans, August 20, 2015, available at macleans.ca/society/health/a-newfound-link-between-brain-injuries-and-adhd.

PART 3: SUSTENANCE OF A BRAIN WARRSIOR

59   Y. Gu, J. W. Nieves, Y. Stern, et al., "Food Combination and Alzheimer Disease Risk: A Protective Diet," *Archives of Neurology* 67, no. 6 (2010): 699–706; and Y. Gu, N. Schupf, S. A. Cosentino, et al., "Nutrient Intake and Plasma Beta-Amyloid," *Neurology* 78, no. 23 (2012): 1832–40.

60   K. A. Dougherty, L. B. Baker, M. Chow, and W. L. Kenney, "Two Percent Dehydration Impairs and Six Percent Carbohydrate Drink Improves Boys Basketball Skills," *Medicine and Science in Sports and Exercise* 38, no. 9 (2006): 1650–58; and M. S. Ganio, L. E. Armstrong, D. J. Casa, et al., "Mild Dehydration Impairs Cognitive Performance and Mood of Men," *British Journal of Nutrition* 106, no. 10 (2011): 1535–43.

61   Y. Ogino, T. Kakeda , K. Nakamura, and S. Saito, "Dehydration Enhances Pain-Evoked Activation in the Human Brain Compared with Rehydration," *Anesthesia and Analgesia* 118, no. 6 (2014): 1317–25; and B. G. Perry, T. L. Bear, S. J. Lucas, and T. Mundel, "Mild Dehydration Modifies the Cerebrovascular Response to the Cold Pressor Test," *Experimental Physiology* 101, no. 1 (2016): 135–42.

62   D. Benton, "Dehydration Influences Mood and Cognition: A Plausible Hypothesis?," *Nutrients* 3, no. 5 (2011): 555–73.

63 P. D. Lindseth, G. N. Lindseth, T. V. Petros, et al., "Effects of Hydration on Cognitive Function of Pilots," *Military Medicine* 178, no. 7 (2013): 792–98.

64 D. Ludwig, *Always Hungry?* (New York: Grand Central, 2016).

65 I. Cusin, F. Rohner-Jeanrenaud, J. Terrettaz, and B. Jeanrenaud, "Hyperinsulinemia and Its Impact on Obesity and Insulin Resistance," *International Journal of Obesity and Related Metabolic Disorders* 16, suppl. 4 (1992): S1–11.

66 R. O. Roberts, L. A. Roberts, Y. E. Geda, et al., "Relative Intake of Macronutrients Impacts Risk of Mild Cognitive Impairment or Dementia," *Journal of Alzheimer's Disease* 32, no. 2 (2012): 329–39.

67 C. S. Souza, B. S. Paulsen, S. Devalle, et al., "Commitment of Human Pluripotent Stem Cells to a Neural Lineage Is Induced by the Pro-Estrogenic Flavonoid Apigenin," *Advances in Regenerative Biology* 2, no. 29 (2015): 244, available at http://www. regenerativebiology.net/index.php/arb/article/view/29244.

68 O. Okusaga, R. H. Yolken, P. Langenberg, et al., "Elevated Gliadin Antibody Levels in Individuals with Schizophrenia," *World Journal of Biological Psychiatry* 14, no. 7 (2013): 509–15; B. Porcelli, V. Verdino, L. Bossini, et al. "Celiac and Nonceliac Gluten Sensitivity: A Review on the Association with Schizophrenia and Mood Disorders," *Autoimmunity Highlights* 5, no. 2 (2014): 55–61; and M. Urban-Kowalczyk, J. Oemigielski, and A. Gmitrowicz, "Neuropsychiatric Symptoms and Celiac Disease," *Neuropsychiatric Disease and Treatment* 10 (2014): 1961–64.

69 C. W. Leung, B. A. Laraia, B. L. Needham, et al. "Soda and Cell Aging: Associations between Sugar-Sweetened Beverage Consumption and Leukocyte Telomere Length in Healthy Adults from the National Health and Nutrition Examination Surveys," *American Journal of Public Health* 104, no. 12 (2014): 2425–31.

70 R. H. Lustig, *Fat Chance: Beating the Odds Against Sugar, Processed Food, Obesity, and Disease* (New York: Penguin Group, 2012).

71 R. H. Lustig, *Sugar: The Bitter Truth* [video], 2009, available at https://www.youtube .com/watch?v=dBnniua6-oM.

72 E. Schmidt, "This Is Your Brain on Sugar: UCLA Study Shows High-Fructose Diet Sabotages Learning, Memory," UCLA Newsroom, May 15, 2012, available at: http:// newsroom.ucla.edu/releases/this-is-your-brain-on-sugar-ucla-233992.

73 R. Agrawal, E. Noble, L. Vergnes, et al., "Dietary Fructose Aggravates the Pathobiology of Traumatic Brain Injury by Influencing Energy Homeostasis and Plasticity," *Journal of Cerebral Blood Flow and Metabolism*, 36, no.5 (2016): 941–53.

74 A. Sears, "Aspartame—Ant Poison, FDA Complaints," available at alsearsmd .com/2007/02/aspartame-ant-poison-fda-complaints.

75 P. Usai, A. Serra, B. Marini, et al., "Frontal Cortical Perfusion Abnormalities Related to Gluten Intake and Associated Autoimmune Disease in Adult Coeliac Disease: 99mTc-ECD Brain SPECT Study," *Digestive and Liver Disease* 36, no. 8 (2004): 513–18.

76 B. Porcelli, V. Verdino, L. Bossini, L.Terzuoli, A. Fagiolini. "Celiac and Nonceliac Gluten Sensitivity: A Review on the Association with Schizophrenia and Mood Disorders," *Autoimmunity Highlights* 5, no. 2 (2014): 55–61, doi:10.1007/ s13317-014-0064-0.

77 M. Hadjivassiliou, G. A. Davies-Jones, D. S. Sanders, and R. A. Grunewald, "Dietary Treatment of Gluten Ataxia," *Journal of Neurology, Neurosurgery, and Psychiatry* 74, no. 9 (2003): 1221–24.

78 M. A. Arroll, L. Wilder, and J. Neil, "Nutritional Interventions for the Adjunctive Treatment of Schizophrenia: A Brief Review," *Nutrition Journal* 13 (2014): 91.

79 P. Whiteley, D. Haracopos, A. M. Knivsberg, et al., "The ScanBrit Randomised, Controlled, Single-Blind Study of a Gluten- and Casein-Free Dietary Intervention for Children with Autism Spectrum Disorders," *Nutritional Neuroscience* 13, no. 2 (2010): 87–100; and H. Niederhofer, "Association of Attention-Deficit/Hyperactivity Disorder and Celiac Disease: A Brief Report," *Primary Care Companion for CNS Disorders* 13, no. 3 (2011): ii.

80 R. Mesnage, N. Defarge, J. Spiroux de Vendomois, and G. E. Seralini, "Potential Toxic

Effects of Glyphosate and Its Commercial Formulations below Regulatory Limits," *Food and Chemical Toxicology* 84 (2015): 133–53.

81 K. R. Fluegge, "Glyphosate Use Predicts ADHD Hospital Discharges in the Health-care Cost and Utilization Project Net (HCUPnet): A Two-Way Fixed-Effects Analysis," *PloS ONE* 10, no. 8 (2015): e0133525.

82 A. Baden-Mayer, "15 Health Problems Linked to Monsanto's Roundup," EcoWatch, January 23, 2015, available at ecowatch.com/2015/01/23/health-problems-linked-to-monsanto-roundup.

83 J. M. Chan, M. J. Stampfer, J. Ma, et al., "Dairy Products, Calcium, and Prostate Cancer Risk in the Physicians' Health Study," *American Journal of Clinical Nutrition* 74, no. 4 (2001): 549–54.

84 A. Weil, "Does Milk Cause Cancer?," March, 30, 2007, available at drweil.com/drw/u/QAA400175/Does-Milk-Cause-Cancer.html.

85 A. Kyrozis, A. Ghika, P. Stathopoulos, et al., "Dietary and Lifestyle Variables in Relation to Incidence of Parkinson's Disease in Greece," *European Journal of Epidemiology* 28, no. 1 (2013): 67–77; and R. D. Abbott, G. W. Ross, H. Petrovitch, et al., "Midlife Milk Consumption and Substantia Nigra Neuron Density at Death," *Neurology* 86, no. 6 (2016): 512–19.

86 E. M. Schulte, N. M. Avena, and A. N. Gearhardt, "Which Foods May Be Addictive? The Roles of Processing, Fat Content, and Glycemic Load," *PloS ONE* 10, no. 2 (2015): e0117959.

87 M. Hyman, *The UltraMind Solution: Fix Your Broken Brain by Healing Your Body First* (New York: Scribner's, 2007).

88 D. O. Kennedy, R. Veasey, A. Watson, et al., "Effects of High-Dose B Vitamin Complex with Vitamin C and Minerals on Subjective Mood and Performance in Healthy Males," *Psychopharmacology* 211, no. 1 (2010): 55–68.

89 C. F. Haskell, A. B. Scholey, P. A. Jackson, et al., "Cognitive and Mood Effects in Healthy Children During 12 Weeks' Supplementation with Multi-Vitamin/Minerals," *British Journal of Nutrition* 110, no. 5 (2008): 1086–96.

90 M. Micallef, I. Munro, M. Phang, and M. Garg, "Plasma n-3 Polyunsaturated Fatty Acids Are Negatively Associated with Obesity," *British Journal of Nutrition* 102, no. 9 (2009): 1370–74.

91 A. M. Hill, J. D. Buckley, K. J. Murphy, and P. R. Howe, "Combining Fish-Oil Supplements with Regular Aerobic Exercise Improves Body Composition and Cardiovascular Disease Risk Factors," *American Journal of Clinical Nutrition* 85, no. 5 (2007): 1267–74.

92 I. Thorsdottir, H. Tomasson, I. Gunnarsdottir, et al., "Randomized Trial of Weight-Loss-Diets for Young Adults Varying in Fish and Fish Oil Content," *International Journal of Obesity* 31, no. 10 (2007): 1560–66.

93 M. F. Muldoon, C. M. Ryan, L. Sheu, et al., "Serum Phospholipid Docosahexaenonic Acid Is Associated with Cognitive Functioning during Middle Adulthood," *Journal of Nutrition* 140, no. 4 (2010): 848–53.

94 M. A. Aberg, N. Aberg, J. Brisman, et al., "Fish Intake of Swedish Male Adolescents Is a Predictor of Cognitive Performance," *Acta Paediatrica* 98, no. 3 (2009): 555–60.

95 J. L. Kim, A. Winkvist, M. A. Aberg, et al., "Fish Consumption and School Grades in Swedish Adolescents: A Study of the Large General Population," *Acta Paediatrica* 99, no. 1 (2010): 72–77.

96 A. Raine, J. Portnoy, J. Liu, et al., "Reduction in Behavior Problems with Omega-3 Supplementation in Children Aged 8-16 Years: A Randomized, Double-Blind, Placebo-Controlled, Stratified, Parallel-Group Trial," *Journal of Child Psychology and Psychiatry* 56, no. 5 (2015): 509–20.

97 R. Kremer , P. P. Campbell, T. Reinhardt, and V. Gilsanz, "Vitamin D Status and Its Relationship to Body Fat, Final Height, and Peak Bone Mass in Young Women," *Journal of Clinical Endocrinology and Metabolism* 94, no. 1 (2009): 67–73.

98 J. C. McCann and B. N. Ames, "Is There Convincing Biological or Behavioral Evidence

Linking Vitamin D Deficiency to Brain Dysfunction?" *FASEB Journal* 22, no. 4 (2008): 982–1001.

99   M. T. Mizwicki, D. Menegaz, J. Zhang, et al., "Genomic and Nongenomic Signaling Induced by 1alpha,25(OH)2-Vitamin D3 Promotes the Recovery of Amyloid-Beta Phagocytosis by Alzheimer's Disease Macrophages," *Journal of Alzheimer's Disease* 29, no. 1 (2012): 51–62.

100 J. S. Buell, T. M. Scott, B. Dawson-Hughes, et al., "Vitamin D Is Associated with Cognitive Function in Elders Receiving Home Health Services," *Journals of Gerontology Series A, Biological Sciences and Medical Sciences* 64, no. 8 (2009): 888–95.

101 R. Jorde, M. Sneve, Y. Figenschau, et al., "Effects of Vitamin D Supplementation on Symptoms of Depression in Overweight and Obese Subjects: Randomized Double Blind Trial," *Journal of Internal Medicine* 264, no. 6 (2008): 599–609.

PART 4: TRAINING OF A BRAIN WARRIOR

102 R. L. Leckie, L. E. Oberlin, M. W. Voss, et al., "BDNF Mediates Improvements in Executive Function Following a 1-year Exercise Intervention," *Frontiers in Human Neuroscience*, December 11, 2014, http://journal.frontiersin.org/article/10.3389/fnhum.2014.00985/full; C. Tonoli, E. Heyman, L. Buyse, et al., "Neurotrophins and Cognitive Functions in T1D Compared with Healthy Controls: Effects of a High-Intensity Exercise," *Applied Physiology, Nutrition, and Metabolism* 40, no. 1 (2015): 20–27; M. Tamura, K. Nemoto, A. Kawaguchi, et al., "Long-Term Mild-Intensity Exercise Regimen Preserves Prefrontal Cortical Volume against Aging," *International Journal of Geriatric Psychiatry* 30, no. 7 (2015): 686–94; and M. A. Fiatarone Singh, N. Gates , N. Saigal, et al., "The Study of Mental and Resistance Training (SMART) Study-Resistance Training and/or Cognitive Training in Mild Cognitive Impairment: A Randomized, Double-Blind, Double-Sham Controlled Trial," *Journal of the American Medical Directors Association* 15, no. 12 (2014): 873–80.

103 J. E. Friedman, C. M. Ferrara, K. S. Aulak, et al., "Exercise Training Down-Regulates OB Gene Expression in the Genetically Obese SHHF/Mcc-fa(cp) Rat," *Hormone and Metabolic Research* 29, no. 5 (1997): 214–29.

104 O. C. Okonkwo, S. A. Schultz, J. M. Oh, et al., "Physical Activity Attenuates Age-Related Biomarker Alterations in Preclinical AD," *Neurology* 83, no. 19 (2014): 1753–60; and D. Head, J. M. Bugg, A. M. Goate, et al., "Exercise Engagement as a Moderator of the Effects of APOE Genotype on Amyloid Deposition," *Archives of Neurology* 69, no. 5 (2012): 636–43.

105 K. J. Gruber, "Social Support for Exercise and Dietary Habits among College Students," *Adolescence* 43, no. 171 (2008): 557–75.

106 C. Press, "Physical Activity May Leave the Brain More Open to Change," ScienceDaily, December 7, 2015, available at sciencedaily.com/releases/2015/12/151207131508.htm.

107 N. Berryman, L. Bherer, S. Nadeau, et al., "Multiple Roads Lead to Rome: Combined High-Intensity Aerobic and Strength Training Versus Gross Motor Activities Leads to Equivalent Improvement in Executive Functions in a Cohort of Healthy Older Adults," *Age* 36, no. 5 (2014): 9710.

108 J. C. Davis, S. Bryan, C. A. Marra, et al., "An Economic Evaluation of Resistance Training and Aerobic Training Versus Balance and Toning Exercises in Older Adults with Mild Cognitive Impairment," *PloS ONE* 8, no. 5 (2013): e63031.

109 R. A. Mekary, A. Grontved, J. P. Despres, et al., "Weight Training, Aerobic Physical Activities, and Long-Term Waist Circumference Change in Men," *Obesity* 23, no. 2 (2015): 461–67, doi:10.1002/oby.20949.

110 J. J. Avila, J. A. Gutierres, M. E. Sheehy, et al., "Effect of Moderate Intensity Resistance Training during Weight Loss on Body Composition and Physical Performance in Overweight Older Adults," *European Journal of Applied Physiology* 109, no. 3 (2010): 517–25.

111 P. Klainin-Yobas, W. N. Oo, P. Y. Suzanne Yew, and Y. Lau, "Effects of Relaxation

Interventions on Depression and Anxiety Among Older Adults: A Systematic Review," *Aging & Mental Health* 19, no. 12 (2015): 1043–55, doi:10.1080/13607863.2014.997191.; J. K. Sethi, H. R. Nagendra, and T. Sham Ganpat, "Yoga Improves Attention and Self-Esteem in Underprivileged Girl Student," *Journal of Education and Health Promotion* 2 (2013): 55; M. Sharma and T. Haider, "Tai Chi as an Alternative and Complementary Therapy for Anxiety: A Systematic Review," *Journal of Evidence-Based Complementary & Alternative Medicine* 4, no. 19 (2015), doi:10.1186/s13643-015-0005-7; and F. Wang, E. K. Lee, T. Wu, et al., "The Effects of Tai Chi on Depression, Anxiety, and Psychological Well-Being: A Systematic Review and Meta-Analysis," *International Journal of Behavioral Medicine* 21 no. 4 (2014): 605–17.

112 T. M. Eijsvogels, A. B. Fernandez, and P. D. Thompson, "Are There Deleterious Cardiac Effects of Acute and Chronic Endurance Exercise?" *Physiological Reviews* 96, no. 1 (2016): 99–125.

113 S. Hood and R. J. Northcote, "Cardiac Assessment of Veteran Endurance Athletes: A 12 Year Follow Up Study," *British Journal of Sports Medicine* 33, no. 4 (1999): 239–43.

114 G. W. Rebok, K. Ball, L. T. Guey, et al., "Ten-Year Effects of the Advanced Cognitive Training for Independent and Vital Elderly Cognitive Training Trial on Cognition and Everyday Functioning in Older Adults," *Journal of the American Geriatrics Society* 62, no. 1 (2014): 16–24.

115 I. M. McDonough, S. Haber, G. N. Bischof, and D. C. Park, "The Synapse Project: Engagement in Mentally Challenging Activities Enhances Neural Efficiency," *Restorative Neurology and Neuroscience* 33, no. 6 (2015): 865–82.

116 S. Wu, S. Powers, W. Zhu, and Y. A. Hannun, "Substantial Contribution of Extrinsic Risk Factors to Cancer Development," *Nature* 529, no. 7584 (2016): 43–47.

117 A. Bauer, J. W. Kantelhardt, P. Barthel, et al., "Deceleration Capacity of Heart Rate as a Predictor of Mortality after Myocardial Infarction: Cohort Study," *Lancet* 367, no. 9523 (2006): 1674–81; and A. Boskovic, N. Belada, and B. Knezevic, "Prognostic Value of Heart Rate Variability in Post-Infarction Patients," *Vojnosanitetski Pregled* 71, no. 10 (2014): 925–30.

118 A. Roy, D. Kundu, T. Mandal, et al., "A Comparative Study of Heart Rate Variability Tests and Lipid Profile in Healthy Young Adult Males and Females," *Nigerian Journal of Clinical Practice* 16, no. 4 (2013): 424–28.

119 J. A. Chalmers, D. S. Quintana, M. J. Abbott, and A. H. Kemp, "Anxiety Disorders Are Associated with Reduced Heart Rate Variability: A Meta-Analysis," *Frontiers in Psychiatry* 5 (2014): 80; and K. I. Jones, F. Amawi, A. Bhalla, et al., "Assessing Surgeon Stress When Operating Using Heart Rate Variability and the State Trait Anxiety Inventory: Will Surgery Be the Death of Us?" *Colorectal Disease* 17 no. 4 (2015): 335–41.

120 C. A. Lengacher, M. P. Bennett, L, Gonzalez, et al., "Immune Responses to Guided Imagery during Breast Cancer Treatment," *Biological Research for Nursing* 9, no. 3 (2008): 205–14; and C. Maack and P. Nolan, "The Effects of Guided Imagery and Music Therapy on Reported Change in Normal Adults," *Journal of Music Therapy* 36, no. 1 (1999): 39–55.

121 B. L. Fredrickson, M. A. Cohn, K. A. Coffey, et al., "Open Hearts Build Lives: Positive Emotions, Induced through Loving-Kindness Meditation, Build Consequential Personal Resources," *Journal of Personality and Social Psychology* 95, no. 5 (2008): 1045–62; and X. Zeng, C. P. Chiu, R. Wang, et al., "The Effect of Loving-Kindness Meditation on Positive Emotions: A Meta-Analytic Review," *Frontiers in Psychology* 6 (2015): 1693.

122 J. W. Carson, F. J. Keefe, T. R. Lynch, et al., "Loving-Kindness Meditation for Chronic Low Back Pain: Results from a Pilot Trial," *Journal of Holistic Nursing* 23, no. 3 (2005): 287–304.

123 M. E. Tonelli and A. B. Wachholtz, "Meditation-Based Treatment Yielding Immediate Relief for Meditation-Naive Migraineurs," *Pain Management Nursing* 15, no. 1 (2014): 36–40.

124 D. J. Kearney, C. A. Malte, C. McManus, et al., "Loving-Kindness Meditation for

Posttraumatic Stress Disorder: A Pilot Study," *Journal of Traumatic Stress* 26, no. 4 (2013): 426–34.

125   A. J. S. T. Farsides, "Brief Loving-Kindness Meditation Reduces Racial Bias, Mediated by Positive Other-Regarding Emotions," *Motivation and Emotion* 40, no. 1 (2015): 140–47.

126   M. K. Leung, C. C. Chan, J, Yin, et al., "Increased Gray Matter Volume in the Right Angular and Posterior Parahippocampal Gyri in Loving-Kindness Meditators," *Social Cognitive and Affective Neuroscience* 8, no. 1 (2013): 34–39.

127   B. E. Kok, K. A. Coffey, M. A. Cohn, et al., "How Positive Emotions Build Physical Health: Perceived Positive Social Connections Account for the Upward Spiral between Positive Emotions and Vagal Tone," *Psychological Science* 24, no. 7 (2013): 1123–32.

128   B. Goldstein, *The Secret Language of the Heart: How to Use Music, Sound, and Vibration as Tools for Healing and Personal Transformation* (San Antonio, TX: Hierophant, 2016).

129   J. Lieff, "Music Stimulates Emotions through Specific Brain Circuits," March 2, 2014, available at jonlieffmd.com/blog/music-stimulates-emotions-through-specific-brain-circuits.

130   C. Grape, M. Sandgren, L. O. Hansson, et al., "Does Singing Promote Well-Being?: An Empirical Study of Professional and Amateur Singers during a Singing Lesson," *Integrative Physiological and Behavioral Science* 38, no. 1 (2003): 65–74.

131   V. N. Salimpoor, M. Benovoy, K. Larcher, et al., "Anatomically Distinct Dopamine Release During Anticipation and Experience of Peak Emotion to Music, *Nature Neuroscience* 14, no. 2 (2011): 257–62.

132   F. H. Rauscher, G. L. Shaw, and K. N. Ky, "Listening to Mozart Enhances Spatial-Temporal Reasoning: Towards a Neurophysiological Basis," *Neuroscience Letters* 185, no. 1 (1995): 44–47.

133   A. V. Nedeltcheva, J. M. Kilkus, J. Imperial, et al., "Sleep Curtailment Is Accompanied by Increased Intake of Calories from Snacks," *American Journal of Clinical Nutrition* 89, no. 1 (2009): 126–33.

134   G. S. Tajeu and B. Sen, "New Pathways from Short Sleep to Obesity? Associations between Short Sleep and 'Secondary' Eating and Drinking Behavior," *American Journal of Health Promotion,* November 11, 2015.

135   L. Harmat, J. Takacs, and R. Bodizs, "Music Improves Sleep Quality in Students," *Journal of Advanced Nursing* 62, no. 3 (2008): 327–35.

136   N. Goel, H. Kim, and R. P. Lao, "An Olfactory Stimulus Modifies Nighttime Sleep in Young Men and Women," *Chronobiology International* 22, no. 5 (2005): 889–904; and M. Hardy, M. D. Kirk-Smith, and D. D. Stretch, "Replacement of Drug Treatment for Insomnia by Ambient Odour," *Lancet* 346, no. 8976 (1995): 701.

137   B. J. Bushman, C. N. Dewall, R. S. Pond Jr. and M. D. Hanus, "Low Glucose Relates to Greater Aggression in Married Couples," *Proceedings of the National Academy of Sciences* U.S.A. 111, no. 17 (2014): 6254–57.

138   J. Jaekel, S. Eryigit-Madzwamuse, and D. Wolke, "Preterm Toddlers' Inhibitory Control Abilities Predict Attention Regulation and Academic Achievement at Age 8 Years," *Journal of Pediatrics* 169 (2016): 87–92.

139   J. Skorka-Brown, J. Andrade, B. Whalley, and J. May, "Playing Tetris Decreases Drug and Other Cravings in Real World Settings," *Addictive Behaviors* 51 (2015): 165–70.

PART 5: ESSENCE OF A BRAIN WARRIOR

140   P. A. Boyle, L. L. Barnes, A. S. Buchman, and D. A. Bennett, "Purpose in Life Is Associated with Mortality among Community-Dwelling Older Persons," *Psychosomatic Medicine* 71, no. 5 (2009): 574–79; R. B. Cohen, C. Bavishi, and A. Rozanski, "Purpose in Life and Its Relationship to All-Cause Mortality and Cardiovascular Events: A Meta-Analysis," paper presented at the Epi Lifestyle 2015 Scientific Sessions meeting of the American Heart Association, March 3–4, 2015, Baltimore, MD; and P. L. Hill and N. A. Turiano, "Purpose in Life as a Predictor of Mortality across Adulthood," *Psychological Science* 25, no. 7 (2014): 1482–86.

141 A. Steptoe, A. Deaton, and A. A. Stone, "Subjective Wellbeing, Health, and Ageing," *Lancet* 385, no. 9968 (2015): 640–48.

PART 6: RESPONSIBILITIES OF A BRAIN WARRIOR

142 M. E. Pembrey, L. O. Bygren, G. Kaati, et al., "Sex-Specific, Male-Line Transgenerational Responses in Humans," *European Journal of Human Genetics* 14, no. 2 (2006): 159–66.

143 D. Zhou and Y. X. Pan, "Pathophysiological Basis for Compromised Health beyond Generations: Role of Maternal High-Fat Diet and Low-Grade Chronic Inflammation," *Journal of Nutritional Biochemistry* 26, no. 1 (2015): 1–8.

144 S. Karsli-Ceppioglu, A. Dagdemir, G. Judes, et al., "Epigenetic Mechanisms of Breast Cancer: An Update of the Current Knowledge," *Epigenomics* 6, no. 6 (2014): 651–64; D. P. Labbe, G. Zadra, E. M. Ebot, et al., "Role of Diet in Prostate Cancer: The Epigenetic Link," *Oncogene* 3, no. 36 (2015): 4683–91; and M. L. Suva, "Genetics and Epigenetics of Gliomas," *Swiss Medical Weekly* 144 (2014): w14018.

145 M. J. Dauncey, "Nutrition, the Brain and Cognitive Decline: Insights from Epigenetics," *European Journal of Clinical Nutrition* 68, no. 11 (2014): 1179–85; and M. Devall, J. Mill, and K. Lunnon, "The Mitochondrial Epigenome: A Role in Alzheimer's Disease?" *Epigenomics* 6, no. 6 (2014): 665–75.

146 O. Babenko, I. Kovalchuk, and G. A. Metz, "Stress-Induced Perinatal and Transgenerational Epigenetic Programming of Brain Development and Mental Health," *Neuroscience and Biobehavioral Reviews* 48C (2015): 70–91; M. Debnath, G. Venkatasubramanian, and M. Berk, "Fetal Programming of Schizophrenia: Select Mechanisms," *Neuroscience and Biobehavioral Reviews* 49 (2015): 90–104.

147 C. Lesseur, A. G. Paquette, and C. J. Marsit, "Epigenetic Regulation of Infant Neurobehavioral Outcomes," *Medical Epigenetics* 2, no. 2 (2014): 71–79; O. Babenko, et al., "Stress-Induced Perinatal and Transgenerational Epigenetic Programming," *Neuroscience and Biobehavioral Reviews* 48C (2015): 70–91.

148 M. A. Reddy, E. Zhang, and R. Natarajan, "Epigenetic Mechanisms in Diabetic Complications and Metabolic Memory," *Diabetologia* 58, no. 3 (2015): 443–55; and W. Yuan, Y. Xia, C. G. Bell, et al., "An Integrated Epigenomic Analysis for Type 2 Diabetes Susceptibility Loci in Monozygotic Twins," *Nature Communications* 5 (2014): 5719.

149 B. G. Dias and K. J. Ressler, "Parental Olfactory Experience Influences Behavior and Neural Structure in Subsequent Generations," *Nature Neuroscience* 17, no. 1 (2014): 89–96.

150 K. Gapp, S. Soldado-Magraner, M. Alvarez-Sanchez, et al., "Early Life Stress in Fathers Improves Behavioural Flexibility in Their Offspring," *Nature Communications* 5 (2014): 5466.

151 B. M. Kuehn, "The Brain Fights Back: New Approaches to Mitigating Cognitive Decline," *Journal of the American Medical Association* 314, no. 23 (2015): 2492–94.

152 Marigold Associates, "Adaptive Change: The Supportive Role of Community," June 28, 2011, available at marigoldassociates.com/adaptive-change-the-supportive-role-of-community.

153 T. Rosenberg, *Join the Club: How Peer Pressure Can Transform the World* (New York: Norton, 2012).

PART 7: YEARLONG BRAIN WARRIOR BASIC TRAINING STARTS WITH THE 14-DAY BRAIN BOOST

154 E. W. Iepsen, J. R. Lundgren, J. J. Holst, et al., "Successful Weight Loss Maintenance Includes Long-Term Increased Meal Responses of GLP-1 and PYY 3-36," *European Journal of Endocrinology* 174, no. 6 (June 2016): 775–84, doi:10.1530/EJE-15-1116.

Index

Crunchiness of food, 46
Crystal, Billy, 39
CT (computed tomography) scan, 65
Curcumin, 129

Daily habits and routines (*see* Training of a
    Brain Warrior)
Dairy products, 85, 126, 133, 135, 161–65,
    261, 264
  glycemic load (GL) for, 116, 118–19
Daniel Plan, 48, 239
Dating sites, 6
Davis, Anthony, 82
Daytime fasting, 137
Decision-making skills, 205–9, 213, 215
Deep-breathing exercises, 222
Defeat, as state of mind, 37
Defense, U.S. Department of, 9
Degenerative nerve disorders, 123
Dehydration, 111
Dehydroepiandrosterone (DHEA) level, 80,
    184
Dementia, 4, 39
  attention deficit disorder (ADD)/
    attention deficit hyperactivity disorder
    (ADHD) and, 8
  beta amyloid plaque formation and, 137,
    172, 189
  brain scans and, 7, 8, 64
  defined, 86
  epigenetics and, 2, 235–36
  fat-free diet and, 123
  omega-3 fatty acids level and, 168, 170
  risk factors for, 87–96
  as umbrella category, 86, 87
Depression and anxiety, 3, 4, 39, 58, 244
  Alzheimer's disease and, 8, 94
  ANTs and, 190–92
  attention deficit disorder (ADD)/
    attention deficit hyperactivity disorder
    (ADHD) and, 8
  brain injury and, 64
  brain type and, 65–66
  dating sites and, 6
  diet and nutrition and, 107
  fat-free diet and, 123
  gut health and, 85
  heart rate variability (HRV) training and,
    193
  herbs and spices and, 132
  incidence of, 8
  low levels of anxiety, 40
  obesity and, 8, 71
  omega-3 fatty acids level and, 124, 168, 170
  pesticides and, 161
  as risk factor for dementia, 87, 93, 94
  serotonin levels and, 141–42
  sleep apnea and, 92
  sleep deprivation and, 202, 203
  sugar and, 148

  untreated, 94
  video game addiction and, 6
  vitamin D levels and, 171, 172
Deprivation mind-set, 38–40
Dessert, 262–63, 306
Detling, Nicole, 197
Detoxification, 81, 113, 129, 184, 317
Diabetes, 3, 4, 15–16, 39, 71, 73
  agave and, 150
  artificial sweeteners and, 152, 153
  consequences of, 9
  diet and nutrition and, 77
  dietary fat and, 124, 126
  epigenetics and, 2, 235–36
  exercise and, 184
  fat-free diet and, 122
  gluten and, 157
  incidence of, 8–9
  laboratory tests and, 75, 77
  as risk factor for dementia, 88
  sleep deprivation and, 202
  sugar alcohols and, 154
  sugar and, 148
  vitamin D levels and, 171
Dias, Brian, 235
Diastolic blood pressure, 74
Diet and nutrition, 15, 94, 99–174, 177
  allergens, elimination of, 135–36
  anti-inflammatory foods, 79
  brain types and, 67
  breakfast, 136, 206, 262, 271, 276, 305
  carbohydrates (*see* Carbohydrates)
  cheat days, 301
  cholesterol levels and, 76
  corn, 135, 160–61, 261, 264
  dairy products (*see* Dairy products)
  diabetes and, 77
  dining out, 142, 147, 206, 277
  elimination diet, 136, 264
  excuses and, 42–43
  fasting, 136–37
  fat-free diet, 122–23
  fats, 4, 102, 122–28, 294
  fiber (*see* Fiber)
  fish and seafood (*see* Fish and seafood)
  focus on abundance not deprivation, 38–40
  folate-rich foods, 79
  food choices, 138–47, 174
  foods to limit or avoid, 147–65, 174, 264
  fruits and vegetables (*see* Fruits;
    Vegetables)
  gluten, 78, 135, 156–59, 165, 261, 264,
    289, 294
  grains, 109, 110, 119, 156–57, 261, 264
  grocery shopping, 144–47
  herbs and spices, 129, 130–32
  in history, 103–7
  human chorionic gonadotropin (hCG)
    diet, 256
  inflammation and, 84

Loving-kindness meditation (LKM),
195–96, 215
Low-density lipoprotein (LDL) levels, 76,
121, 125, 126, 129, 148
Ludwig, David, 115
Lunch, 262–63, 271, 305
Lunchables, 45
Lustig, Robert, 148
Lymphoma, artificial sweeteners and, 153

Maca root powder, 289
Macadamia nut oil, 128
Magnesium, 69, 205
Maltitol, 155
Maltodextrin, 151, 158
Maltose, 151
Mandela, Nelson, 11, 219
Manganese, 150
Mangosteen, 112
Maple syrup, 150
Marijuana, 89, 90, 95, 202, 203
Marshmallow test, 209
Martial arts, 11–12, 17, 37, 60, 220–21,
225
Martin, Leslie, 57
Massachussets Male Aging Study, 83
Mayan cultures, 160
Mayo Clinic, 122
McDonald's, 47
McGill University, 141
Meadowsweet, 131
Meat, 85, 125, 126, 135, 139, 142, 146
Medical hypnosis, 94
Medical marijuana, 89
Medications, 8, 86, 130–31, 133, 166, 167,
202, 251–52
Meditation, 69, 74, 94, 96, 105, 193, 205,
215, 223, 224
loving-kindness meditation (LKM),
195–96, 215
Melatonin, 205
Meltiness of food, 46
Memory, 43, 82, 88, 92, 94, 111, 132, 137,
143, 170
Menopause, 203
Menstrual cycle, 141
Menstruation, 79, 80
Mental exercise, 188–89
Mental health issues, 64, 65
Mental rehearsal, 198
Mental workouts, 60
Mentors, 20, 224
Metabolic syndrome (MetS), 78, 88, 150,
152
Metabolism, 112, 132, 136, 153, 183–85,
294, 318
Methamphetamines, 44
Microsoft, 6
Military service, obesity and, 9
Milk, 116, 161–64

Mind-set of Brain Warriors, 17, 25–53
changing focus on dietary changes, 38–40
churches and, 47–49
examples of, 29–30, 50–52
fast track versus incremental approach,
18–19
food advertising and, 44–46
identifying as healthy person, 34–37
knowing purpose, 30–34
mass denial and anxiety levels, 40–41
mechanical phase, 19, 21–22
primitive phase, 19, 20–21
spontaneous phase, 19–20, 22–23
takeaways, 53
wolves, sheep, and sheepdogs, 27–28
Mindful exercise, 184, 186
Mischel, Walter, 209
Mistakes, learning from, 24, 57, 198–99,
208, 210–11, 215
"Moderation, everything in," 24, 34
Mokolo (gorilla), 108–10
Molasses, 151
Moldy: The Toxic Mold Movie
(documentary), 251
Mongols, 105
Monosodium glutamate (MSG), 135, 143
Monounsaturated fat, 125
Morphine, 44
Moskowitz, Howard, 44–45
Motivation (see Mind-set of Brain Warriors)
MRI (magnetic resonance imaging), 65
Mullen, Admiral Mike, 230
Multiple sclerosis
artificial sweeteners and, 153
pesticides and, 161
vitamin D levels and, 171
Multivitamins, 167–68, 177, 260
Music, 199–201, 215
mybrainfitlife.com, 70, 180, 195, 199, 204,
205, 260, 262
Myelin, 198
Myristic acid, 126

Naltrexone, 165
Naps, 204
Native Americans, 106, 133, 160
Nature, 192
Neurofeedback, 231
Neurons, 90, 143
Neuropathy, 90, 124
Neuropsychological test, 70
Neuroscience, 5
New England Journal of Medicine, 238
New learning, 187–89
New York Times Magazine, 45
Newcastle University, 88
News outlets, 5–6
Niacin, 76
Nicotine, 44, 83, 203
Nighttime fasting, 137, 306